Waiting to Hear
"Momma"

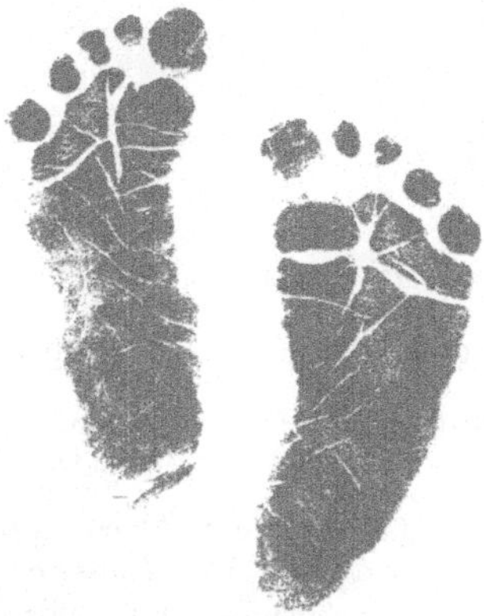

Waiting to Hear "Momma"

A MOTHER'S MEMOIR

Lucille Messina

Waiting to hear "Momma" A Mother's Memoir

Unsuccessful attempts were made to track down the copyright owners of "Footprints in the Sand" and "Heaven's Very Special Child" poems.

For information about this title or to order other books and/or electronic media, contact the publisher:

SpecialChild Press, LLC
SpecialChildPressLLC@gmail.com

Library of Congress Control Number: 2019903354

ISBNs:
Softcover: 978-1-7336662-0-6
Hardcover: 978-1-7336662-2-0
eBook: 978-1-7336662-1-3

Printed in the United States of America

Cover and Interior design: 1106 Design

What if your child could never say "Momma" or your child could never say "Daddy"?

This compelling true story chronicles a mother's faith and unconditional love journey through fear, anger, deep depression, guilt, loneliness, and discrimination while caring for her special child. As a reader, you are transported into the highs and lows encountered in the healthcare system, government, and business world as they impacted their lives. It tells how this mother was thrust into a world that she never knew existed, where doctors were not gods who could fix everything.

Waiting to Hear "Momma" is a memoir by a mother of a special child who finds herself struggling to survive. The yearning of a mother to hear "Momma" is deep and emotional, with a bond that goes beyond the spoken word. Communication can be non-verbal and sometimes sealed within, where only two people in the entire world speak the same language.

"The world breaks everyone, and afterward, some are strong at the broken places."

—Ernest Hemingway

To my husband, Karl: You are my rock that held our family together. I dedicate this to you, because without your love, patience, devotion, and logical approach, our family could not have survived. You are one in a million.

Acknowledgments

I would like to thank the following, who guided and supported me to finish this memoir.

Erika Duncan and the Herstory Writers Workshop, for the countless hours helping me realize the importance of being in the moment that I often missed and pushing me back to a place I never wanted to relive. Meredith Rawls Favicchia for your honesty and support. Joan Hogan for informing me about the workshop, the months of editing and being a sounding board for my ideas. Geraldine McNeela for your critiques and encouragement. Karl Messina for being my partner in this journey and for recalling moments that I'd suppressed. Marytheresa Messina for being my first critic and the first who shed a tear. Valerie Spatola for your review and finding the right word when it seemed impossible. Finally, Amy, for being the light at the end of the dark tunnel.

As the mother of a special child, I would like to extend my deepest appreciation to the doctors and nurses who sincerely tried to make our lives better in the face of often-insurmountable obstacles.

I wish to thank Manatt, OPWDD and St. Mary's Healthcare System for Children for gathering the information and creating the "CHILDREN AND YOUNG ADULTS WITH MEDICAL FRAGILITY: A Population Needs Assessment."

Contents

Prologue

The bathtub is filling up with warm water, and Jacklyn is lying on her side, enjoying the soothing and caressing warmth of the slow-rippling flow. Her eyes are wide open as she listens to the whooshing sounds coming from the faucet. I'm giving her a bath as I focus on her back and the curve that is twisting her body. My fingers run along her spine as if I could mentally transform this bend into a straight line. I carefully wash her beautiful auburn hair, making sure not to get a single drop of shampoo into her eyes. At eight years old, she has grown to fill more than half the length of the tub.

After a few minutes, she seems uncomfortable but cannot verbalize her distress, so I interpret in ways others do not understand and place the wash towel on her pale shoulders to give her extra warmth. I analyze her every movement, every facial and bodily signal. She raises her fisted hands to her face and appears to be soothed while uttering a low grunt. I kiss her cheek and say, "I love you" before lifting and wrapping her thin frame into a large towel. She has put on weight, and I'm glad for that, but I know each lift becomes more concerning. Next, I cradle her in my arms to give her my own body heat as we both sit on the bathroom floor. Meanwhile, this gives me a moment to rest my arms, back, and legs, hurting from the strain. Now, as I am rocking her in my arms, I think back to the transformation from a naïve mother to who I have become today.

"We know what we are but know not what we may be."

—William Shakespeare

Sweeping the Clouds Away

Karl was off to work, and I was starting to get accustomed to the routine of being a new mother—a mother of a beautiful baby girl. It was still hard for me to wrap my mind around the fact that I was a mother, that I had a baby to raise, to teach, to love. She had completed us; we were a family, to enjoy boundless hours of wonder and delight. Jacklyn would soon be four months old. I reviewed the *TV Guide* for children's shows and was pleased with the future possibilities my baby would enjoy. *Sesame Street* was on the top of my list, followed by *Muppet Babies, Fraggle Rock, Thomas and Friends, Mister Rogers' Neighborhood,* and *Reading Rainbow.* Today, we cuddled while *Sesame Street* was on TV, and I read her nursery rhymes. While pinching each toe, I chanted, "This little piggy went to market, this little piggy stayed home . . ."

She fell asleep after her morning bottle. I was content just holding her in my arms. I was utterly mesmerized by her. Her soft wrinkles, folds of chubby skin, and rosy cheeks—a true gift from God. I inhaled with my lips on her forehead, trying to breathe in all of her. She smelled so fresh, a floral and vanilla scent, with such tiny hands and feet. She had the darkest of auburn hair, upon which I could already place a small hair clip.

It turned out to be a bright, crisp winter morning, so I decided to place Jacklyn in her playpen before tackling chores: doing our laundry, catching up on housecleaning, and writing thank-you notes for many of the baby gifts kept me occupied. I located my Aunt Carol and Uncle Tony's gift of a white, blue, and orange Raggedy Ann doll and placed it over the playpen, so Jacklyn could see it. She stared at it for an hour!

The next day was January 12, 1985, and it started out as a chilly weekend. A bit of frost covered the lawn. Karl and his brother Ken had planned to go cod fishing off Long Island. It was a simple pleasure that they both enjoyed from childhood. He left around 4:00 a.m. as I wished him good luck.

Later in the morning, I fed Jacklyn breakfast before searching her closet for a new outfit. First, I started flipping through the top rack, and then I started on the second row. Finally, happy with my decision, I chose the red corduroy pants and white turtleneck sweater with multi-colored hearts on it. I brushed her dark auburn hair up into a tiny little pony tail and placed a matching multi-colored heart Velcro hair tie to secure it. She smelled like baby powder, and her skin felt satin soft and new. I admired and caressed her tiny toes before putting ruffled white socks on her feet. All this was happening as we could hear the *Sesame Street* theme song "Sunny Day" playing in the next room. I loved to sing to her this happy tune.

The melody ended, and, while she was still on the changing table mat, something happened. Her face changed to a grimace, her skin turned blue, and her eyes twitched. The contortion of the right side of her little face was more intense as I watched in horror. "Jacklyn, Jacklyn!" I yelled, but she was unresponsive. She appeared not to be breathing during this episode. The wind knocked out of me, I froze. Feeling faint, my hands clenched the table. I started to tremble uncontrollably, my stomach turned—something was very wrong. I laid my hand over her tiny chest while gasping for air.

I don't know how many seconds or minutes passed. Her normal color and breathing returned. I rushed and called my mother-in-law to get word to Karl out at the dock when the boat returned to shore. My mother-in-law calmly told me that I should go directly to the hospital. Her cool composure settled me down just enough to act. I picked up Jacklyn, grabbed the diaper bag, and ran out the door to my car. I found myself constantly looking in the back seat to make sure she was conscious and breathing. I prayed that I would not get into an accident. I repeated the Hail Mary and Our Father. My body felt numb, and I don't remember physically driving my car to the children's hospital.

There I was, standing at the emergency room door, as Jacklyn was transported onto a hospital bed while I was asked numerous questions. Within seconds, she was rushed past a room filled with waiting patients. A team of doctors surrounded her to the point that she was obscured from my sight. I paced back and forth until I noticed Karl rushing into the room. He was disheveled; his hair was matted down with perspiration, and his fishing jacket was filthy. Fear was clearly evident on his face.

As the hospital's team prepared for Jacklyn's admission, I felt like I was watching a movie—not part of the script, isolated, and alone. Doctors and nurses appeared to be moving back and forth in slow motion. Numbness and denial took hold of my body. Within hours my life had been turned upside down. What had just happened to my baby?

I watched as Karl filled out paperwork and talked to the hospital staff. He looked shaken, occasionally glancing my way. His eyes had a wild, glazed look I'd never seen until today. My husband—my rock, never rattled, always calm in any situation—was not the same man.

Trying to calm myself, I thought, *We are in a very good hospital with excellent doctors, and they will fix whatever problem has developed. Since I'm a new, inexperienced mother, I probably didn't properly handle my newborn correctly. Maybe she had an allergic reaction to something, or maybe I was mistaken, and she was just having a difficult bowel movement. She has been eating well and gaining weight, and, therefore, this is just a panic attack on my part.* I reassured myself that everything would be resolved and back to normal very soon.

The hospital released her after days of tests and said her EEG was normal but that her eyes were not tracking objects. We needed to follow up with various doctors in the next few weeks. I had to be patient and have complete trust that the future visits would set things right.

During the next few days, I did not see another episode. My daily routine to observe her tracking objects was relentless—to the point I thought I was going insane. Yes, she was, no she wasn't, then yes, then no. At times, my face would be an inch from her eyes as I looked intently, searching for the slightest movement or reaction—until I didn't know if I was truly witnessing something or if my imagination was playing tricks on me. One day, after more attempts, I tried to relax and erase the frightening thoughts that were racing through my mind—terrifying visions of her future. Resting my head on the kitchen table, I closed my eyes. I started to float back to the carefree days when I was pregnant—those lighthearted days, filled with innocence and lofty expectations.

I thought back to the summer of 1984. We'd attended all the Lamaze classes, and I started to think about my own delivery. I did not handle pain well, and the prospect of an episiotomy depicted in the video shown in class scared the hell out of me. Karl was calm and supportive every day, with a Rubik's Cube being his favorite source of relaxation.

I was surprised with a baby shower and was overjoyed with the adorable baby toys and clothing. At the shower, my niece Roseann conveyed her personal childbirth experience to me. She said it would be like having bad cramps—certainly reassuring news for me to hear. During the following weeks, my worried emotions eased with the anticipation of such a precious gift as I felt this new life kicking within me. Seeing my baby's movements as I curiously watched my belly ripple and move from within was like a dream coming true.

The nursery was near completion. The oak changing table, dresser, and canopy crib had been delivered. A teddy bear theme for the nursery was perfect. The musical mobile, crib blanket, lamp, and wall décor all had a brown bear dressed in a striped pink, green, blue, yellow, and white nightshirt and matching hat. Placing the cute big brown bear wall décor, with its comforting eyes, was important to me. I positioned it right over our baby's bed, so it would be a calming sight when our little one looked up. I dreamed of our child's first steps, recitals, Disney trips, first word, school plays, and on and on. Our newborn, the expression of our love, would be here soon.

I read that the first child arrives later than predicted. I was naïve; my water broke two weeks earlier than expected. I don't know if all my nesting activities caused this to happen, but I'm sure cooking trays of lasagna to freeze for the planned christening didn't help. I wasn't packed for the hospital. That was unusual for us because, as a couple, we planned for everything. Overhearing Karl's conversation with the doctor's answering service, I could tell we had to wait until the office was open. We quickly packed an overnight bag, and then I returned to the bedroom. After another contraction, I heard Karl starting to mow the lawn. *What is he doing? He's crazy! How could he time me?*

The pain was extreme, and I wasn't handling it well. It was a warm day, and the windows were open as the fresh air filled the room along with the smell of newly cut grass. An hour passed, and we finally were on our way to the doctor's office as I sporadically punched the ceiling of the car with each excruciating abdominal cramp. Karl confessed to me that he was timing my contractions as he mowed the lawn. He could clearly hear my screams of pain from *outside* the house—over the noise of the lawnmower!

The doctor's waiting room was crowded with mothers-to-be and their families. They were exchanging small talk while some children played with each other. All the seats were occupied, and there was a lively mood in the air. I quickly rushed into my doctor's office without screaming. The timing was just right. The doctor's longtime assistant carefully guided me into the exam room. Upon examination, I was informed it was time to head for the hospital. After I dressed, a tremendous wave of pain hit me. "Give me something! Give me something!" I yelled and screamed. I continued requesting pain medication as I was hunched over and repeatedly punched the exam table with my fists. After the pain subsided, I turned and realized the exam room door was open for everyone to hear me roar.

As Karl helped me to the car, we had to pass through the waiting room again. This time I took notice of all those happy young mothers-to-be I had seen earlier. Now, it was dead silent, and each of these ladies had buried their faces in the various magazines they provide in a doctor's waiting room. I didn't see anyone's face as I exited the room. No one uttered a sound or looked at me, and for that, I was thankful. All I

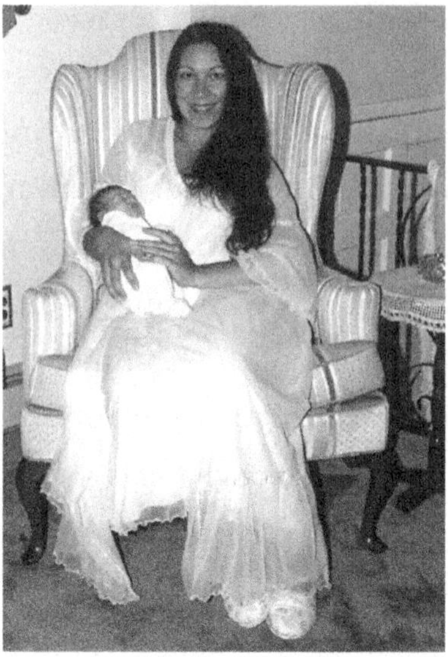

kept sensing was that this experience was not going to be "just bad cramps," as my niece Roseann suggested. She'd hardly had any pain—three pushes and she was done.

After eight hours of labor, Jacklyn was born on September 25th. Choosing her name was a work of art. I picked "Jack" to honor my father, who had passed many years prior. Since my father-in-law was named "Jasper," it was also fitting and honored him as well. I added "lyn" to put the finishing female touch to it.

Arriving home with our new baby was joyous. My hopes and dreams had come true. Karl and I gladly shared our funny moments of the event with all our friends and family visitors. Life was good.

"Just Pray She Is Only Blind"

We spent countless hours attempting to witness Jacklyn track objects; finally, we made an appointment to have her eyes checked at the children's hospital. Within weeks, Jacklyn had numerous eye tests taken, and we had a follow-up arranged to hear the results. As we sat in the waiting room, I watched the other children playing. I started to notice some differences. The babies sat up, turned, and grabbed at toys that their older siblings were holding. I thought, *Jacklyn is just low key compared to the other children. All babies have different temperaments; Jacklyn is just quiet and calm. She doesn't fuss or cry a great deal. I'm a lucky mother to have such a tranquil child.*

We finally were called into the office. The doctor said he detected clinical delays and that her vision response test was abnormal. He also indicated that the EEG was normal at the point in time it was taken. This did not mean she did not have a seizure disorder. He spoke about delays in development; but, as a new mother, I was oblivious as to what the doctor was alluding to. Maybe I was hearing only what I wanted to hear.

The folder we brought that contained the recent medical data now had additional notes from Karl regarding this visit. Upon exiting the office, Karl safely tucked this growing stack of papers into his briefcase. He paused as we were leaving the hospital's front entrance and turned to me. His facial expression was different, not like anything that I had seen before. Looking into my eyes, he said that I should ". . . just pray she is *only* blind!"

I felt like someone had punched me in my stomach, but it was just Karl's bluntly delivered way of waking me up to reality. Shocked, I sensed myself slipping, descending into a dark hole. Mentally, I needed a wall, one so high that no negative comments from Karl or anyone else could reach me. Alone in my own little private world, all the terms discussed earlier by the doctors came back to me in images—of her alone, walking with a cane, of her in a wheelchair, of her shaking violently from a convulsion. The awful terminology I'd previously dismissed flashed past in dreamlike visions, as if I were on a merry-go-round: going around with no way of getting off. I saw the frightening pictures over and over again with each turn. Nevertheless, I held on for dear life, clutching the pole on the horse to keep me from being thrown off.

We drove home in silence. That night, I made dinner, with Karl's help, but all I could remember was how red wine can dull a horrible pain.

Jacklyn was put on phenobarbital to manage any seizures. Weeks passed, and we found ourselves back in the hospital for the second time because her seizures had become uncontrollable. The medicine was *not* working! The seizures were brief—lasting less than one minute. Sometimes it appeared as a noticeable startle or a very scared look on her face and her arms stiffening. Other times they were more violent, with her entire body jerking upward and her face twitching. I had witnessed her seizing every few minutes until she fell asleep. Her body was exhausted from the one to ten daily episodes. With every seizure I witnessed, a little piece of me died. Each time, it added another brick to the wall that was growing higher to shield me.

The hospital's neurologist entered Jacklyn's room and started reviewing her charts. He decided to change her medication to control the convulsions. I asked him what other kinds of tests could be done, and his response was to "bring her back in two years if she is still alive." Staring at him with my mouth open, I was speechless.

What did he just say to me? My mind raced, and it struggled to make sense of what had just happened. *This can't be true.* As her parents, we were both healthy, and nothing in our families would have indicated any problems. I even had an amniocentesis because of my age. I couldn't move, transfixed, still staring, while the doctor walked out of the room. Now horrific visions flashed before my eyes as I found myself leaning on Karl, who was at my side.

This was the beginning of the mourning I felt over the loss of a healthy child. I felt an overwhelming sense of doom of what now *could* be my daughter's future in contrast to what it *should* have been. My dream shattered into pieces. Each milestone, each anticipated moment that should have been joyful was falling before me, now broken and crushed into fragments of her life's potential. There had to be a reason and a solution—and I needed to know what it was, very soon, before it was too late.

An Early Intervention preschool program was offered to us during this most recent hospital visit. I eagerly took advantage of the program, as this intervention would help her in range of motion and sense of balance, and it would help drain excess mucus from her lungs. Since she was missing visual stimulation, it would help her get on track. I received a phone call from a physical therapist who was assigned to Jacklyn's case. We made an appointment for the following week.

It was a chilly morning, around 10:00 a.m., and Jacklyn had a light breakfast. She was six months old and unable to sit up. I was instructed not to overfeed her because the therapy session might upset her stomach. She had been experiencing reflux, and we didn't want to cause her any more distress.

Avoiding the seriousness of the situation, I started searching her closet for a cute outfit. I dressed her in a new, beautiful pink-and-white dress and white tights—just one of many gifts she'd received. She looked like a little doll as I put the finishing touches on my precious baby girl. A little pink hair clip in her auburn hair that matched her dress was all I needed to complete the job.

Karl was at work, and I was anticipating Jacklyn's first therapy session. This intervention was unquestionably going to help her. My hopes and expectations for the therapy was the much-needed boost that would extinguish my fears and give Jacklyn the best opportunity to overcome her illness.

As I held Jacklyn in my arms, I glanced out the window and saw a car pull up. They were on time. Two young ladies, one blonde, the other brunette, exited the car with two large bags of equipment. They entered the house and introduced themselves as Alice and Cheryl. I offered them refreshments. I was in hostess mode since we'd had many friends and family visitors over the past few weeks. They declined and proceeded to ask questions and jotted down notes.

Next, they requested that I remove her new pink dress and put her in a loose one-piece outfit. Cheryl said many parents make this mistake and don't realize exactly what is involved during a physical therapy session. My mood changed soon after satisfying her request. I watched as they placed her over a large ball to give her vestibular stimulation. They explained it would help her sense of balance.

Next was postural drainage. By getting her in positions and then gently "clapping" her chest, it would make it easier for mucus to drain from her lungs. I tried to learn and took some notes, but it became too much for me to see—too much for me to accept. Removing myself, I walked into the kitchen. I needed to visualize what the future would be when she improved. Then, with clenched fists, I fantasized about baby play dates as most new mothers would be experiencing now, only to be summoned back by Cheryl requesting extra cloths—"to soak up drool and reflux discharge." Re-entering the room with the extra towels, I was forced to see Jacklyn draped over the large rubber ball, struggling to raise her little head. Her tiny arms were next to her chest as she tried desperately to push up while they cheered, "Come on, Jacklyn—you can do it!"

Alice and Cheryl made routine visits. They suggested a beanbag chair for her, and we quickly purchased a beige one.

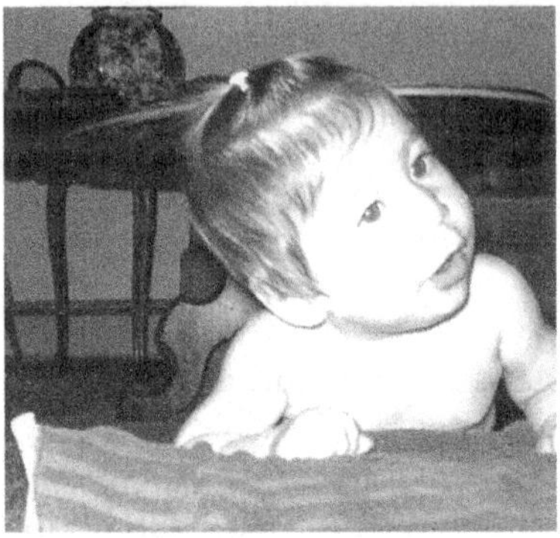

It became her comfy chair; it helped with the postural-drainage therapy and was a source of alternative seating. Jacklyn was turning nine months old, and I learned how to keep her lungs clear, help her sense of balance, and what type of tactile stimulation would be useful. It was not unusual to have feathers, furry pieces of material, and sandpaper, just to name a few, as tactile objects next to her beanbag chair. I was optimistic and felt their knowledge and support would make a difference in Jacklyn's life.

One Saturday morning after breakfast and after months of therapy, Karl and I placed Jacklyn on a mat to try to get some sense of her accomplishments. We placed her on her stomach, and, to our surprise, she pushed and held her head up.

We started cheering and yelling, and she rolled over. It might have taken her longer, but she achieved rolling over by herself. I couldn't wait to tell everyone and write about this milestone in her journal.

EEG Results

Jacklyn's seizures had been in control—now, it seemed, *she* had the upper hand over *them*. I was on an emotional high, almost dizzy with happiness to see her push up on her tiny arms and then roll over. I was yelling, *"Look, Karl, look at her, look, yippee Jacklyn, yippee, keep going, wonderful job, my little peanut!"* Karl and I were elated and cheering her on. He ran to the phone and started calling his parents to tell them the great news. I could hear him shouting, "She pushed up and rolled over." As he was about to make another call, I hollered for him to hurry back into the room.

Karl stood in the hallway, grasping the railing, and his proud grin changed. Our happiness was short-lived, as a bout of seizures followed. Her teeny arms jerked upward above her head, collapsing at her side. At the same time, it propelled her chest upward, while her top lip pressed down and moved in one direction and the bottom lip went the opposite way. A red to almost bluish color overshadowed her face, and her eyes were squinted, almost shut. As her face twitched, she seized repeatedly. I watched, helpless and discouraged, while waiting for the doctor to return our call. The crushing weight on my chest from panic pushed all the air from my lungs as I picked Jacklyn up, wrapping my arms around her and holding her close. I placed my outstretched fingers over her little head and gently rubbed, wishing I could magically erase this disease that had trapped her.

"Please, God, through my fingers, send a cure." I sobbed, "Jacklyn, it's going to be okay. Mommy and Daddy are here." Finally, her doctor called with detailed instructions on a medication change.

The seizures subsided. Jacklyn, exhausted from the episode, was resting. My adrenalin pumping, I became angry and focused on the inevitable consequences it would have on Jacklyn as she got older. She was just a baby now, but what would happen as she matured and the physical therapy and seizure medication did not help? I became angry at the doctors who were not rectifying what appeared to be many painful seizures. I became angry—at God, too. I was a good, church-going person, so why me? Why my baby? I even became angry at myself. I was a failure. I failed to produce a healthy child. Soon all my anger turned to fear. Fear for her future. Fear for our new family and the marital stress that could develop.

Within a few days, she was placed into the hospital for additional tests. It was late on a Friday afternoon that I sat quietly waiting for her to recover from the anesthesia. Karl was at work, anticipating my call. It was getting dark, as evening was approaching. The adjacent rooms were vacant, and the entire hospital floor was strangely silent. Our room was dark, with only a small overhead bed light shining. The brightness from the adjacent parking lot lamps cast an eerie glow through the slanted blinds. I could see the attending nurse at the large reception station outside our room. Patricia was slender, with short, sandy-brown hair, and little makeup. She appeared to be alone handling the desk duties.

The metal guardrails on Jacklyn's bed were up. They looked huge in contrast to her tiny body; she had absolutely no ability to move them. Our nurse checked on Jacklyn and asked me, "Do you need anything to make you more comfortable?"

"Thank you, no," I replied. Then I asked, "When will the doctor see us with the test results?"

"I'll find out," she responded.

Mentally, I kept reassuring myself that everything was going to be fine. I had to hold on and believe. I comforted myself by whispering, "Relax. Keep calm. I must have faith because I'm in one of the best hospitals in the area, with the best doctors."

A long time passed, and finally a young, tall, red-haired doctor entered the room. Expressionless, he strolled directly over to the hospital bed as I stood up to greet him. I was optimistic but soon felt flushed with fear as I grasped onto the cold, silver metal railing of Jacklyn's bed. Surely this could not be more grave news. He introduced himself to me and then stated, "Her brain waves are abnormal. Her life expectancy will be short, probably only a few years."

With this, I started to shake.

He continued by saying, "Didn't anyone explain this to you?" He seemed agitated. I stared at him and attempted to speak but no words came out. I continued to shake, but now I was shaking so badly that the guardrails I was holding started to clang loudly. He then stated, "I have prior dinner plans with my wife and have to leave." He promptly made an about-face and walked away, passing that nurse, who was still at her work station.

The clanging from the rails continued and was now loud enough to echo in the empty room. Soon, Patricia, our nurse, appeared with a cup of water. She slowly peeled each finger of my left hand and then my right off the long railing. She had a sympathetic touch, holding both my hands, squeezing them gently while gradually backing me into a side chair next to Jacklyn's hospital bed.

As my body was trembling uncontrollably, she looked into my eyes and asked, "How are you and Jacklyn getting home?" She continued to speak to me gently and asked if I needed her to call someone to assist me.

Finally, I said, "My car is somewhere in the parking lot." With her assistance, I telephoned Karl. He was at work, a few miles away.

Waiting for Karl to arrive, I thought, *My child looks so peaceful, covered in the crisp white hospital sheets.* My mind wandered. I imagined her in a little white coffin, in a white lace dress with ruffled white ankle socks. The glowing rays of light that surrounded her were blinding me. *No, no! I can't allow that to happen. It had to be me instead, not her, not her. Please God, take me!* Sobbing, I buried my face into my lap.

As Karl entered the room, Patricia approached him. They talked briefly before she handed him some paperwork. Karl's face was pale, and his eyes looked at me with concern and tenderness. He picked up Jacklyn, who was coming out of the anesthesia, gently patted her back, and kissed her. "Let's go home."

In the days that followed, I sensed how fortunate I was to be married to this man, as I lounged in bed longer than necessary, unable to start my day. I started to reminisce about my life to that point. I mentally wanted to transport myself back to another time and place.

The incident with the callous doctor delivering the EEG result to me still played out in my mind. The sound of the shaking guardrails continued to echo in my head. *Clang! Clang! Clang!* I fell asleep at night only to twitch each time I relived that moment. I was stuck somewhere between denial and acceptance, but my desire to give Jacklyn the best chance was unyielding. It was the only thing driving me. An opportunity for that was created by a recommendation to change her neurologist. I jumped at the prospect. The new hospital was located about one hour from our home in eastern Long Island. I planned to stay overnight with her in preparation of early-morning tests.

Driving up to the hospital building, I noticed it appeared strikingly taller in comparison to the surrounding structures. I parked and removed our belongings without waking Jacklyn up. She had just fallen asleep. Staring at her little face, so innocent, I loved how the sun reflected the red highlights in her auburn hair. They sparkled like bits of glitter sprinkled from a fairy godmother's wand. As I headed toward the elevator, I broke out in a cold sweat, my palms tingling. A loud voice in my head kept saying, *What if you get more grave news and another doctor like the last one?*

Soon we settled into a private corner hospital room. Jacklyn woke up with a small seizure—the face that was so sweet looking just half an hour ago was now twisting and turning red. It was a small, short-lived seizure, and she came out of it quickly. Holding her close, I told her, "It will be fine, my pretty girl. They will fix you." Kissing her cheek, I whispered, "This is a getaway weekend for you and Mommy." I started playing her music box to fill the air with a happy sound to cover the beeping medical equipment just outside our door.

As Jacklyn and I settled into the hospital room, her new neurologist entered. She was a small woman, about five feet tall, with short blonde hair and soft brown eyes. She introduced herself and started to discuss in detail Jacklyn's upcoming tests and prognosis. I tried to comprehend. I shook my head. It felt like she was speaking a foreign language. *What is wrong with me? I'm not right!*

"I'll speak to your husband when he arrives tomorrow," she stated in a soft voice while patting my shoulder. *Does she really see me—this shell of a person that is Jacklyn's mother?*

After she left the room, I wanted someone to fix Jacklyn at any cost. I wanted to hear only good news. *Maybe it will be this doctor and this hospital!* I was thankful that night to have a new doctor with the insight to see me for what I had become. I sensed she was far from a cold, detached physician. As I unpacked, a nurse gave me an extra food tray and asked if I needed anything. "No, this is perfect. Thank you," I replied. The food tray was a thoughtful gesture. Kindness and understanding by those who welcomed me at this new hospital was the best medicine, and it didn't cost anything.

During the night, I had trouble getting into a comfortable sleep position in the reclining chair. I found it impossible to turn from side to side. My back hurt—but not as much as the awful thoughts racing around in my head. It is there that the burden of anticipation regarding the next day's schedule was weighing heavily. I prayed my rosary, asking that the answers to fix my child would soon be found.

Still being a novice to this routine, I decided to sleep on the wide windowsill instead of the recliner. Granted, it was a bit cold and hard, but sufficient. I had a clear view looking down at the people entering and leaving the main entrance. We were in a unit on one of the top floors of the hospital. I noticed a family with a young child exiting with balloons and fantasized that we would be happily leaving soon.

"Hello. Excuse me," the nurse said as she entered our room. "I need to give Jacklyn her meds." I nodded and gently lifted her into my arms while watching the nurse perform her duties. A syringe filled with liquid seizure medication was placed into the corner of Jacklyn's mouth, followed by a slow push on the cylinder tube.

Kissing Jacklyn good night, I covered her with a blanket and tucked a pillow at her back and legs for support. I opened her music box for one final tune to play out before lowering the lights. Slowly I walked back to my windowsill bed, and thought, *How wise to have windows that did not fully open!*

I fell into a deep sleep, free-falling downward, spinning faster and faster as I was transported somewhere else in time, drifting and escaping the present.

Early-morning rays of sunshine woke me with warmth, touching my cheeks. The new day felt bright, but my windowsill bed had left me with aches and pains. Moving slowly, I checked on Jacklyn, and she was still asleep. Soon a teenage hospital volunteer entered. Becky had a spare breakfast food tray and offered me the meal. I thanked her. The hot coffee was weak but hit the spot. She told me she was a new volunteer. Her shift had ended, but her mom couldn't pick her up for another hour. She also confessed that her boyfriend, also a new volunteer, had just started his shift. She wasn't in a rush and asked if I wanted company. She looked melancholy, and I sensed she was troubled. I decided to ask her what was wrong.

"Oh, it's boyfriend problems," she replied. Then she asked me, "How did you find your husband?"

Pressing my lips together, I looked at her, so young, bright-eyed, with a fresh innocent view of the world. I was like that so many years ago. As we continued, I asked if she really wanted to know the full story.

"Yes, please," she replied. Escaping the present seriousness that brought me here, I recalled my early days—my first marital mistake, my second chance, and then, miraculously, a dream come true. I spilled out my life as if I wanted to prepare her for some of the challenges the future might hold.

For the next forty-five minutes, she listened as I recalled my past, beginning with childhood memories that transported me back to the days when I was a young girl—much younger than Becky. Like many young girls, I would play dress-up in a pretend white wedding gown and marry. This would be followed with baby dolls, bottle feeding, and diaper changing. As I grew from a child to an adult, I desired a career but never lost the passion to have a family.

My parents were dedicated, loved each other, and worked as a team. To me this was a relationship I yearned for. Yet on September 2, 1982, I faced the stark reality of my current situation. I found myself sitting in a divorce lawyer's office as I rehashed in my mind how I'd gotten to this point in my life, especially being Catholic—and the only one in my immediate family who was a divorce statistic.

I was basically a gullible and soft-hearted person. A bit sheltered as a child, I always believed people were responsible and trustworthy. That was then, but this turn of events propelled me to become stronger and wiser. I had to take charge and follow my dream of someday having a family. My soon-to-be-ex-husband admitted, *after* we were married, that he did not want children. For me, this was grounds for divorce. The annulment would take some time, and I already had the paperwork at home to review. I drew strength from recalling my grandparents' enormous sacrifice to have a better life in America. The decisions they made were hard but necessary for them to reach their goals. I felt empowered to act and start anew. This was a setback, but I was determined it would not affect my lifetime vision.

My attorney sat behind his large cherry wood desk and started reviewing the divorce paperwork. He was an older man, small in stature, with a receding hairline. I found his advertisement in a local newspaper, quoting a low price for simple divorces. His office was neat, plain—not one that a prominent lawyer would occupy. Brown wooden panel walls and dull décor was the theme of his office. He did not have a secretary, and he handled all the documentation and transactions by himself. Nevertheless, the simple no-fault divorce was signed, sealed, and delivered to me, and I handed over my check in final payment for his services.

After visiting my attorney on that Friday afternoon, I spent the entire weekend working on my annulment. This was unfinished business if I wanted to be married in a Catholic church. It turned out to be more emotional than I imagined and a revelation on my part. As an independent woman, I had to be strong. There are steps in life that help define your maturity, and I realized that weekend that my decision was truly the right one toward my personal growth. I matured far more in a brief period than I could have ever imagined.

This was a wake-up call on the road of life. The only thing fouler would have been the lack of action on my part and a loveless marriage. Being truthful to your spouse and oneself is priceless. It's part of one's character and upbringing. I've learned that mutual goals, honesty, and respect would carry a relationship. Making an excuse and not facing the facts will lead only to disaster. Hopefully, my dream to have a future with a family could still come true. The following Monday, I arrived at work legally a free woman.

I learned a tremendous lesson in life. Starting to date again was scary. I was determined not to be fooled again. Before long I noticed eligible and potential men to date, but no one really interested me. Months passed, and I became more involved with projects at work as well as overseeing my mother's needs now that my father was gone. She was the typical Italian mom—always making sure you had enough food. She never learned how to drive. My attempt to teach her on my father's red Ford almost landed us on a neighbor's front lawn.

One day, a newly hired young man named Karl started working in my office, and we had been assigned a few projects together with other team members. I needed his expertise on various technical problems I was having, and he obliged. His blue eyes were clear and bright. He had golden brown hair and a ruffled beard. I soon found myself attracted to him. We started to date, and I learned he was kind, patient, honest, understanding, and the most logical person I had ever met. He was smart and could communicate well at all levels of the business world, from bikers, all the way to presidents and CEOs of companies. I thought he was one in a million as well as a good cook, too. He had an Italian, Irish, and German background with qualities that were distinctive of each culture. He loved to dine at nice restaurants, and we did that often.

Since I was the older person in this relationship, I was concerned about our future. I wasn't going to make any more mistakes. He left the company to explore other opportunities, but we continued to date. I discovered that an age difference of seven years did not matter. I did find it amazing that we had the *same* birth month and day. We had similar values and goals, and we respected each other. A bright future was ahead of us, and we were ready to make a life and family together. I hoped for a positive result as I waited patiently for the verdict from the church officials, looking forward to a new life spiritually and emotionally. Within a few months, I received my annulment. Karl proposed, and we married. Just over a month into our marriage, we learned I was pregnant.

One of the many beautiful things about finding true love is when you realize you want to give that special person everything. Having a family together is the greatest devotion and complete self-giving experience a couple can have. Life was good, and we were looking forward to making our dreams come true.

"Well, Becky—that's my story," I confessed.

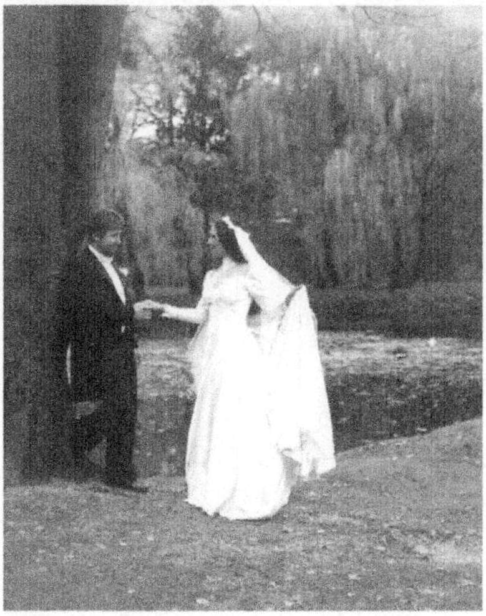

"Thank you very much for sharing it with me. I hope to see you tomorrow," she replied and gave me a long goodbye hug. I softly patted her back and then tossed her long hair off her face. Almost one hour had gone by, and Becky hadn't said one word during that time, but her expression told me all I needed to know. Her surprised, wide-eyed, innocent look reminded me of myself in my younger days. Being there in the hospital with Jacklyn and not knowing what was coming left a big hole in the story. For now, though, I thought she'd heard enough!

Returning to Work

The last EEG did not provide any hopeful news. We'd had her tested by numerous other doctors. Meanwhile, my maternity and extended medical leave ended, and, physically, I was ready to return to work. Karl and I had discussed this many times, and he was wise to realize I had to return to work to help my mental state. The road I was going down was a slippery slope, and this was the only choice.

Sleepless nights were common for me, but the night before heading back to work was different. The fear of facing Penny, Mary, Lorraine, Jason, Dan, and Jennifer—all their questions and my explanation all played out in my mind. What would I say? How often would I have to explain something I didn't want to talk about or even believe was real? Could I just say everything was fine, knowing they would obviously see past my lie? I was never good at hiding my true feelings for a long time. They eventually would discover the truth. All they would have to do is look into my eyes to see the pain. My stomach started to hurt as I faced the fact that I had to return to the same location where, not long ago, I was surrounded with happy faces, baby gifts, and good-luck wishes.

I dressed that morning in a plain gray business suit. The color matched my emotions. Karl was still asleep, but Jacklyn was awake. Her eyes were wide open, and she was listening intently to every little sound that could be heard so early in the morning. Maybe she was focusing on the birds chirping outside or the noise I made in preparation for my day. She appeared uneasy, possibly sensing my anxiety. Comforting her, I gently kissed her cheek and whispered, "I'll be back soon—love you." I tucked the blanket around her before leaving the house to go to the train station.

As I parked my car at the station, my stomach continued to ache, making me realize I'd made a wise choice not to have eaten breakfast. Knowing my niece Roseann would be over later to babysit Jacklyn gave me little relief. My distress was mounting with each passing block that distanced me from home.

It was a short thirty-minute ride to the office. Boarding, I avoided sitting with anyone I had befriended through the years. I moved from car to car to escape detection, almost like a thief trying to get away from being captured by the officials. Yes, I had a price on my head, with my picture on the wanted poster. It said, "WANTED: Terrible Mother"; "WANTED: Mother Who Leaves Her Sick Child." Yes, I was guilty—guilty as charged. Lock me away, long enough for this bad dream to vanish. Jacklyn had become my greatest joy and my greatest sorrow.

Quickly exiting the train at my destination, I moved at a rapid pace down the damp, musty stairway to the lower street level that was filled with foul odors. Miraculously I avoided any eye contact with associates during the short walk to my office.

Fortunately, my cubicle was near the front door. I went directly to my desk and started to obtain the necessary passwords to reestablish access to our computer system. Sitting in the high-back office chair was as close to being hidden from the world as I could get right now. I wished I were a smaller person and that the chair were wider and higher, hiding me from all eyes. Being quiet as possible with little movement, like a mouse attempting to escape detection, was my best option. There was no other place to run or hide. Oh, to be invisible for just a few hours until I could figure out how to cope! I continued to keep my back to the passing traffic until someone noticed me as they walked up and down the aisle. Then, I was greeted with a sympathetic smile and an occasional soft-spoken "welcome back."

Jason was the first person who sat down in the one small guest chair that fit in my cramped cubicle. His gray hair highlighted the well-known fact that he had personally experienced life's low point with illness in his family. Speaking with a somber expression, he cut the formalities short and said that I "had a tough road ahead of me." He confessed that he'd heard from a reliable source about Jacklyn's condition. He called her "Jackie." This was the first time my child had been called "Jackie," and it felt like he was talking about another baby, not mine! In an odd way, I wished that were true.

A reliable source had told one co-worker, so, therefore, others—or maybe everyone—knew! Who was that source? Who did I convey my deepest thoughts to while I was on maternity leave? I started to have flashbacks to when Karl was away on a business trip. The phone rang one evening, and it was Jennifer, a co-worker who had taken over my tasks while I was on leave. She needed advice on an office turnover procedure. I was in the kitchen, an almost-empty bottle of Merlot sitting on the oak kitchen table. Circles on the brown wood from the dried-up spilled red wine were near my wine glass. *Yes*, I recalled. I had been talking to Jennifer, and the more wine I drank, the more I talked and cried to her. I explained how Karl had said, "Just pray she is *only blind*," and how the doctor said, "Bring her back in two years if she is still alive." As I emptied my heart and soul, I emptied the bottle, too. She certainly was the source who'd exposed me.

I continued listening to Jason's words of wisdom and wondered if my eyes looked as sad as the eyes of this man, who was thirty years my senior. My head was swimming with thoughts, concerns, and fear that I could absorb only so much of his advice. He then got up, wished me luck, and left my cubicle to attend a meeting. Afterward, I wondered if I should have asked Jennifer not to divulge Jacklyn's condition. It wasn't her fault, and I certainly couldn't change the past.

Pity was not the emotion I wanted from anyone, nor did I want to feel different from the families of my co-workers. But my family was different. Now, the detachment and feeling of alienation I had struggled with was weighing on my shoulders with a vengeance. The thought entered my mind that I should just give up and go home. Karl would be disappointed. Deep down inside, I knew that I had to overcome this first day because it represented the first day of the rest of my life as a working mother of a special child. I had to keep those wine bottles corked and my emotions sealed.

The initial months were a sequence of stressful adjustments to find the right medicine and dosage. On one occasion, while my niece was caring for Jacklyn, she called me; and, with urgency in her voice, said Jacklyn was seizing repeatedly. I had only minutes to react and make the next train home or wait almost another hour. I grabbed my bag and started running for the train. I was in panic mode.

At certain stations, every time the doors opened, we lingered longer than usual for passengers to exit the car. I had to control myself from yelling at them to move faster. *Why is the engineer driving this train so slowly? Why do we have to make a stop when not one passenger gets off or on the train?* The conductor's crackly voice filled the car from the overhead speakers: "The next station will be Floral Park." Every passing minute, I wondered if my niece had to call 911. Would I be too late—had they already left for the emergency room? Finally reaching my stop, I rushed to my car. Driving the half-mile home, I used back streets, avoiding any main roads and traffic lights.

Within five minutes of entering the house Jacklyn had another seizure, her face turning red and twitching, her little arms jerking upward and then coming to rest at her side. As I watched her, the feeling of helplessness was overwhelming. How I wished it could be me! Immediately I called and left a message with her neurologist.

Patiently waiting for the return call, I held Jacklyn in my arms as my niece looked on with deep concern. We both were scared. She was nervous and apologized for not being able to handle the situation. I didn't blame her and said, "You did the right thing." Jacklyn was damp from sweat, her mouth slightly open, with drool running down the left side of her little cheek, sleeping, exhausted from the episode. She was no longer flushed, and her breathing had returned to normal. I wondered how much damage these seizures were causing and if they could be stopped with new medicine.

I don't recall how many minutes passed, but the neurologist called with a plan that included a medication change. I placed the additional phenobarbital liquid into a syringe and gently placed a few drops at a time into the side of her mouth, making sure she received it without coughing or aspirating. Slowly, I continued until the syringe was emptied. Next, writing down the doctor's instructions in detail, I waited and observed to see if the additional medicine was taking effect. Still cradling her, I called my direct boss regarding my current situation and that I would make up the time in the following days. Finally, I remembered to take a breath of air into my lungs and stop the dizziness, the hyperventilating. Time passed, with no additional seizing. I sat in silence with my body shaking, thinking I'd made it through this one this time! We'd both survived.

Thankfully, the following week was uneventful, yet I had to be ready at a moment's notice. I never knew when I answered the phone if it was a life-or-death situation or a user from another department requesting technical support.

One morning, I observed a different assistant at the front desk. Our paths had crossed before during my employment, and we cordially greeted each other. We both belonged to a women's professional network. It was a rough road for all women in the business world during this time. She approached me that day when no one was within hearing distance and totally surprised me with her confession. Her shocking reveal was to the point. She'd overheard a few supervisors declaring they wanted to get rid of me because of the difficulties I was having at home. I wouldn't be any good to them in the office with my family health distractions.

Her statement hit me and hit me hard. I'd been blindsided, and I was horrified. She continued with her paperwork, so as not to draw attention. I gave her a nod, whispered "Thank you," and continued with my duties. During the remainder of the day, I repeatedly found myself shaking my head. What more could be thrown at me? At the same time, I started to wonder if there could be a double standard in my workplace.

How callous and cruel to find myself in another fight to survive. Yes, this was another battle, a different type of war. I knew the disease and how to counteract that assault. There wasn't an unknown entity attacking me—only those in charge, who had not walked in my shoes. I was tired, so very tired, and I thought, *Will I have enough strength to march forward and defeat yet another enemy?* It was near 5:00 p.m., so tomorrow would be another day and another skirmish in my never-ending wars.

Heading to the train station on my way home, I noticed a young high school boy carrying a book on Julius Caesar. I recalled a high school class assignment where we discussed Shakespeare's *Julius Caesar* and how he was surrounded by his enemies. Treachery destroyed Caesar's will to live; his final words were "*Et tu, Brute*?" as he was stabbed. I, too, felt sharp-bladed knives at my back—the cutting words I'd just heard. Being isolated, surrounded, and attacked can and will defeat you if you allow it to happen. All my years of dedicated service were not going to be ruined by a few callous people. I was not going to allow this to happen, especially as a woman in today's business world. I had to fight and fight hard for myself and my family. Any change in our medical coverage would affect Jacklyn's care. Her treatment was my primary concern. Increased financial burden and additional marital stress were also at stake.

As I sat on the train heading home, the only plan I could think of was to keep detailed notes to counteract every accusation with my own claim. It was a start, and at least they would know I wasn't going to take this lying down.

While keeping my journal of daily issues I was experiencing heartburn, abdominal pain, and reflux. The daily burning pain and discomfort in my throat became unbearable. Not one of the over-the-counter relief medications I carried with me was doing the trick. My physician instructed me to get an upper

GI endoscopy. Fearful of being watched and judged, I didn't want to take off from work and bring any more attention to my problems. Desperate, and with very few scheduling options, I arranged a lunchtime procedure at a hospital near my office to be done *without* anesthesia. As the flexible hose was placed into my mouth, I closed my eyes. Relax; then swallow; relax; then swallow, until the tube hit its mark.

Waiting for the technician to finish, I thought about those past few weeks and the human capacity for burden. Was it human nature to get rid of the ugly, the distasteful, the unpleasant, and want around us only the perfect, happy, and successful? Foolish are those who are not compassionate and understanding, because it is rare to find someone who has not been exposed to hardship in their lives. It happens to all of us; it is just a matter of time until someone's own dark cloud appears overhead.

Baby Photos

Fighting management was another job on my plate. But, for that day, I had to continue to survive; I had to jettison what was out of my control, this navigating who is my friend or my foe. That day-to-day office stress had to be locked in my mental file cabinet for another time because I was home now with other obstacles in my path.

Leaving the sanctuary of our home was a big step I had to take to belong and be part of our community. I craved the connection to other young mothers and feared that Jacklyn would be isolated. She could be set apart and not have contact with other children. I had to break out of our comfort zone before it became a prison.

The holidays were approaching, and I wanted a traditional holiday photo of Jacklyn to give to family and friends. I dressed her in a new green velvet dress with white lace trim collar and white tights. Admiring my efforts, she looked perfect for her scheduled holiday photo shoot. I put her hair up and placed a large towel that was made into a bib under her chin, so her dress and coat would stay clean. I'd learned to keep extra towels on hand for her unexpected reflux, which often had a terrible odor.

Our high ranch-style house was not ideal for the logistics of our new reality, and getting down the fourteen steps of our home with Jacklyn in her custom-made chair was always a challenge. I strapped her body and legs into the large, foam body-support insert and slowly started to wheel her down each step inside the house, expressing happily, "Pretty girl, my little sweet pea, here we go." *Slow and steady*, my inner voice repeated. *Slow and steady, very slow and very steady!* The right wheel and then the left; to the second step. Then the right wheel, followed by the left wheel; now I was on the third step. I was scared and worried. What if she had a seizure? I had to sit down on a step while holding onto the chair handles, my head lowered, my arms outstretched, my hands sweaty, until I could rally enough willpower and continue onto the interior landing. I tried not to, but it was impossible not to contemplate how I could manage this as she grew and gained weight.

Finally, I reached the landing. I thought to myself, *Wow! Halfway there!* Next, I had to open the front door and maneuver the outside seven steps to the driveway. The weather was always a factor, but I could not let it stop me. Rainy days were the worst, and today happened to be one of them. I attempted to grasp an umbrella, but it was ludicrous to hold an umbrella while performing such a task. I placed a plastic tarp over her to shield her from the deluge until I reached the car. *Here I go again—slow and steady—down each step.* While the rain saturated my hair and coat, it was a small price to pay to keep her dry.

As I drove into the underground parking lot, I noticed there was no available handicap parking. I drove around the lot once, twice, and by the third time, a woman entered a car which opened a large spot near the entrance to the department store. This allowed me enough space to get the body-supporting chair and Jacklyn out of the car. By this time, the moisture from the rain had fogged up all the car windows and my eyeglasses. The pain in my back told me how much of a struggle it was, but I managed as a cool breeze helped to refresh me. I gave Jacklyn a kiss and said, "My pretty baby, we are taking holiday pictures of you today." I knew she probably didn't comprehend what I was saying, but her facial expression changed, her eyes widened, and her mouth opened. Seeing her positive reaction to my happiness and excitement gave me more fuel—much-needed energy, when I was so close to empty. It recharged my motherly determination.

As I rolled into the building, I noticed another mother with her children heading for the photo department. *Maybe I'll get a chance to talk to her while we wait our turn.* I briefly stopped to change Jacklyn's bib because it was soiled. She was having a difficult day holding down food. This oversized bib that covered most of her coat was now filled with Jacklyn's breakfast. Then she had a mild seizure. This mother started to stare at Jacklyn. She continued to stare and stare. I became uncomfortable and felt my face flush with alarm. As she was rolling her baby carriage with her two other children walking alongside her, I noticed her outstretched hand shielding their view of Jacklyn. She covered their eyes as she directed them away from our approach. I was enraged, and, at the same time, my heart was broken. My insides were torn to shreds. *Was Jacklyn so terrible to look at? Why?* I asked myself repeatedly. My daughter was as beautiful as any of her children. This could have been a teachable moment for her family.

Yes, Jacklyn was different, but I thought to myself, *Don't ruin this experience for us because of that mother's ignorance.* My motto has always been "Do unto others as you would have them do to you." That day, I didn't get the same respect.

As we entered the photo studio, I removed Jacklyn's coat and wiped any noticeable drool from her face. Luckily this callous mother was not in the waiting room. My eyes were constantly darting toward the entrance, wondering how I would handle a face-to-face meeting if she entered the studio. *Do I verbally attack her, or do I sit quietly and say nothing?*

While waiting to be called by the next available photographer, I viewed the beautiful portraits placed on the wall displaying their professional skills. Most of the children had beautiful smiles in standing and sitting positions while holding a toy or seasonal prop. I hadn't thought this through to that extent, and I started to feel sick to my stomach. Fortunately, the wait time was brief, and we entered the back room.

The staff was kind and realized Jacklyn would be more challenging to obtain that perfect picture every parent strives for. She couldn't see any of the cute stuffed animals the photographer held that would quickly get a reaction, nor could she sit or stand up by herself. Each attempt only produced an unpleasant picture. In the first one, she appeared to be reclining and tilted back so far that her dress exposed too much of her legs. In the next one, she appeared sprawled sideways. With my hair still dripping from the rain and perspiring from my effort to help get that ideal picture, I was drained but still determined. Soon I suggested that, if I placed the prop blanket over my hand and supported Jacklyn from behind, a pleasing photo could be created. I realized this was the only option as I stretched to keep out of the camera's view. With the first few attempts, I was clearly in the photo. I twisted my torso and extended my arm to the extreme. Every one of the muscles along my back, arm, and hand burned with pain. Eventually my distorted body escaped the camera.

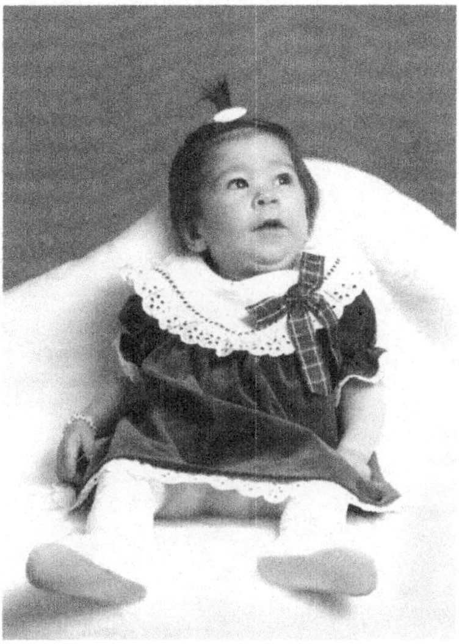

I was content with the pictures taken but also hurt to witness how my daughter could be rejected in this world. I said with a quaver in my voice, "Pretty girl, we're heading home now to see Daddy." I said very little after that for fear she would sense or hear again the tremble in my voice. I was thankful she couldn't see the tears that filled my eyes.

Toy Store and Christmas Gifts

Here it was—an experience I had been dreaming about for years: buying my child Christmas presents in a toy store. Growing up, I might have been told this was where elves stored their handiwork for Santa. As I matured, it always felt like a magical place, allowing children to dream and play in their own fantasy world. My first Christmas with Jacklyn had been joyous, but I was ignorant as to what was to come.

Now, as Jacklyn's second Christmas approached, she was fifteen months old. As I arrived at a huge toy store, I could feel the excitement in the air; however, it was overshadowed with my impression that I didn't belong. I felt like an outsider from another world as I walked masked among the crowd. I was not like the other mothers with healthy children. Jacklyn was different, and the fear of what her future might bring made me shudder. I started to sweat. I opened my coat but still felt the perspiration running down my forehead.

I slowly walked up and down the aisles of the store, only to continually stop, pick up a toy, and say to myself, *No, she can't. My child can't hold that rattle, she can't smile at the cute stuffed bear, can't stand up to play at an art easel, and she can't see the pretty colors on that mobile.* Seeing all the other parents happily shopping with long lists in their hands stirred me up to the point I wanted to yell at them. My inner voice kept screaming, *Don't you realize how fortunate you are to have a healthy child?* I glared at their happy faces as they pushed shopping carts filled to the brim while holiday music played throughout the store. My insides were being torn to shreds with each aisle I walked down and came up empty-handed. I was miserable in a place that gives joy and laughter to so many.

An hour or two passed. I pictured a Christmas tree with no baby toys under it—only clothing, necessities, and physical ther-

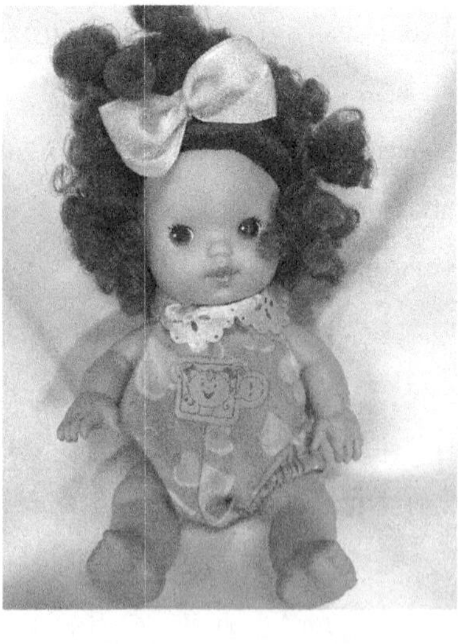

apy items. I started to repeat my search, going down the same aisles again. This time, high on a top shelf, was a small box that contained a four-inch plastic doll with big, curly brown hair, green hair bow, and a white lace collar. She was wearing a one-piece outfit with yellow, pink, and green hearts. This little package was wedged between two much larger dolls. Immediately I thought I could tickle Jacklyn by brushing the doll's hair along her cheek. Upon closer examination, the sticker on it read PRESS HERE. I felt a tiny button under its shirt near its belly. I gently pressed. In a low, childlike voice, it said "Momma." My eyes filled up as I pressed the button again and again.

The satisfaction I got from just hearing that simple word—this small word that I ached to hear—was priceless. I thought, *This milestone in any child's development is usually written in a baby's journal as soon as it is expressed.* I certainly would call family and friends with the desire to tell the entire world of the event. I would make a video and treasure each viewing. I would if only I could! If only I could!

As I headed to get in line with my single purchase, I noticed a baby's "First Year" journal near the register. I'd received a similar one more than a year ago, at my baby shower. But, mine had only the first page completed: Baby name, weight, length, delivery doctor, delivery date, delivery time, and hospital. I hadn't filled in any other pages. There would be few, if any, journal entries for my daughter's accomplishments—so very few!

As I waited patiently for the carts ahead of me to be emptied, I realized my purchase didn't feel so small anymore because we both got a very special present that holiday! Somehow, Santa's little elves knew just what to do.

Group Counseling

We were invited to attend group counseling by Jeanie, a social worker. The holiday season appeared to be the perfect time to start this group. I briefly met her at the hospital and felt a connection because of her compassion and understanding. My expectations were high that this session would help me, reduce my loneliness, and help me feel connected to other families. I pictured a friendship, sort of a bond with other mothers, getting together, having play dates with our special children, sharing and supporting each other like an extended family.

Jeanie, our group facilitator, greeted us dressed in a blue business suit and her dark hair tightly secured into a bun. She directed us to a large conference room not far from the main entrance. Entering, I noticed the white vertical blinds were closed for privacy, and, next to the large brown rectangular office table, was complimentary coffee, water, and soda bottles. Gradually other couples filed in and took their seats.

While waiting for the meeting to start, there was an awkward silence, interaction almost nonexistent. I eyed the other families to get some sense and emotional connection before we started. The couple next to us appeared younger, and the husband had his arm around his wife as they quietly talked. Across from us was an older couple who kept to themselves while drinking coffee.

Jeanie thanked everyone for attending and asked us all to be seated. She instructed us to introduce ourselves and briefly explain our child's medical problem. She indicated to the couple on our left to start and then continue clockwise. After taking a sip of water, the young, disheveled mother started to explain that she was heartbroken because her daughter might lose the sight in her right eye. I didn't want to be cold-hearted, but I thought to myself, *Gee—that isn't a big problem.* The next mother had a son who was in a car accident and lost his leg. The remaining stories were somewhat tragic, but nothing so terrible that I wouldn't trade places with them. I listened while I looked down, so no one could see my eyes rolling with frustration. My face flushed with anger while my hand tightened to the point of almost crushing the coffee-filled Styrofoam cup in my hand. *Damn, I came to this meeting for comfort and support. What the hell am I doing here?*

The more they confessed their misfortunes, the more I felt like a callous monster, just a cold-hearted creature void of sympathy and compassion for their hardships. *This is not me. What have I become?* I was outraged, irate at Jeanie, too, for inviting us, wishing I could run out the door.

It was now my chance to speak. Taking a deep breath, I was still filled with resentment and ashamed at the person I had turned into. In a faint voice, I started by making clear that we didn't have a diagnosis for our fifteen-month-old; Jacklyn was not seizure free, could not see, walk, or talk, and currently was stuck at a one-month developmental level. After I finished, I felt the piercing stares. It was followed by a long, long silence until the social worker started to speak, but I didn't hear anything she said because I was too numb. It was little consolation to me that the other families might have realized their places, their rankings, because no one wanted to win an award here. I secretly wished I could give my "First Place Ribbon" for my hardship to someone else.

After this gathering, I wanted to tell Jeanie how infuriated I was but didn't want to cause a scene. *This confrontation should be done in private when or if I ever get the courage.* How could I question her professional choice or the purpose of this combination of families? One thing for sure was that I left furious and heartbroken. *How could she do this to me? Were we the token "worst case" family to help bring up everyone else's spirits?* This totally rocked my expectations, but I pulled from deep within and hoped other counseling would be different.

We went to various group counseling sessions. Eventually we stopped going to them because we *always* ended up being the worst case. It was causing me more harm than good. I was losing control of my own self-worth, my soul, my essence, my mind. Questions were flying around, over and over, haunting questions that made me constantly place blame on myself.

What did I do to cause Jacklyn to turn out this way? What did I eat? What did I drink? What was I exposed to before and during my pregnancy? I believed this was my fault because I had carried her and must have done something wrong.

In my desire to heal Jacklyn, I tried to negotiate a deal with God: "I would give her my eyes, so she could see; I would give her my legs, so she could walk." I was afraid, so very afraid for her and myself and started to attend healing Masses with Jacklyn while seeking spiritual guidance.

The first healing Mass I attended with Jacklyn was held in a Gothic-style church with beautiful stained-glass windows, dark wood benches, and marble statues. As I carried her in, I was surprised by the crowd. The first ten pews were almost filled, but we found a seat in the fourth row near the aisle. Most of the attendees were older, some with walkers or canes. A few were teens and young adults. I looked around at all their faces. They all seemed to have one thing in common: a peaceful look or maybe an acceptance of the burden they had been dealt. Looking down each row, some held rosaries in their hands, while others just gazed at the altar that was adorned with pink and white flower filled baskets.

Jacklyn had fallen asleep as I gently removed her coat. I admired her resting. She looked like any other baby, with soft, rosy cheeks, chubby legs, and auburn hair pulled up with a Minnie Mouse hair bow. The woman next to me, who was caring for her elderly mom, asked about Jacklyn's problems. After I'd explained, she said, "After tonight she will be seizure free." I reacted with a quivering smile and thought, *How I wish that would come true.* The Mass was brief and was followed by each afflicted person and their caretaker approaching the altar.

Does everyone here think they will be healed? I thought as the pews emptied. I doubted but then felt afraid to doubt, because if I disbelieved, then it might not happen. I tried to shut down that part of my mind, to block the negative thoughts. My gut feelings started to kick in with all their logic and common sense. An internal battle was going on because I so desperately wanted to believe. I thought that miracles do happen, so I prayed, "Please, God, grant this one." This struggle within me continued as I left the church altar immediately after Jacklyn received her special blessing.

I didn't sleep well that evening. Morning came too quickly, and the sun trickled through my peach-colored drapes. I wanted and prayed to see a miracle today. As I slowly turned my body to get out of bed, my right hand hurt. The rosary, still in my hand, had left an imprint of the cross in my palm.

If I don't see a miracle soon, then what can I do next? Where do I turn? Have I become irrational? Am I going crazy? I know I'm slipping, and it's hard to stop. My depression was like quicksand—the hole was getting bigger, engulfing me, and I was falling deeper into it. I wanted my insides to stop throbbing, so I searched for relief in a spiritual way. I came across two poems that had given me some consolation; I'd been reading them almost daily. The poems were "Footprints in the Sand" and "Heaven's Very Special Child."

Footprints in the Sand

One night a man had a dream. He dreamed he was walking along the beach with the LORD. Across the sky flashed scenes from his life. For each scene, he noticed two sets of footprints in the sand; one belonged to him, and the other to the LORD.

When the last scene of his life flashed before him, he looked back at the footprints in the sand. He noticed that many times along the path of his life there was only one set of footprints. He also noticed that it happened at the very lowest and saddest times in his life.

This really bothered him, and he questioned the LORD about it. "LORD, you said that once I decided to follow you, you'd walk with me all the way. But I have noticed that during the most troublesome times in my life, there is only one set of footprints. I don't understand why when I needed you most you would leave me."

The LORD replied, "My precious, precious child, I love you and I would never leave you. During your times of trial and suffering, when you see only one set of footprints, it was then that I carried you."

Heaven's Very Special Child

A meeting was held quite far from earth,
"It's time for another birth,"
Said the Angels to the Lord above,
"This special child will need much love."

Its progress may seem very slow,
Accomplishments it may not show,
And it'll require extra care
From the folks, it meets way down there.

So, let's be careful where it's sent,
We want its life to be content,
Please Lord, find parents and teachers who
Will do a special job for you.

They will not realize right away
The leading role they're asked to play,
But with this child sent from above
Comes stronger faith and richer love.

And soon they'll know the privilege given
In caring for this gift from Heaven.
Their precious charge, so meek and mild,
Is Heaven's Very Special Child.

Friend at Work

Going to work became a much-needed escape and therapy. The personal commitment to tasks at the office continued to provide me with self-satisfaction. I had control and realized my accomplishments daily, whereas, at home, I felt helpless. As I entered my office, I slipped into another dimension like in a science-fiction story. It was like walking through a portal in time and space, where work was the only place I had power over the outcome—a place where mistakes could be fixed and flawlessness achieved. I was transformed into another person; perfection in my work gave me a strange high, and rechecking my work became the norm.

Every day came with different challenges, but coffee breaks and lunchtime were the perfect times for me to let my guard down. I would transform back to the worried, broken-hearted mother who was searching for an answer that would cure her child. As I peeled away the layers to expose my deepest feelings,

Penny was there to listen and advise. She was a unique friend and special co-worker.

One morning, after a terrible weekend of emergency room visits for Jacklyn, I found myself in Penny's cubicle. Thankfully a full tissue box was nearby. The soft white tip of the tissue that was sticking out, peeking from the box top, was calling me. It was such a small object—but one that would absorb my tears, not judge me, and be there for me to get me through another day. Today my nerves were frayed, I had tears in my eyes, and I was extremely depressed, more than usual, unable to escape into any other time or space. There was no place to rest my mind from the internal torture. My heart had been torn to shreds, just like my dream. I was in a fog, hallucinating the "what should have been" for my baby, dreaming and wishing someone would shake me to wake up.

We spoke for a long time while drinking our coffee. Soon, Penny looked into my eyes. I could see her eyes filling up. She reached for my hand; gently holding it, she spoke in a soft voice. "It's time for you to consider seeing a professional counselor." Instantly, it felt like having icy water thrown in my face. I shook my head, trying to wake up from the emotional and mental hole I was digging. My body was trembling, yet it felt like I had a ton of bricks on my shoulders. My chest was heavy from the unreleased tension I held inside. *So, this is how it feels, the weight of truth.* She handed me the tissue box and said, "You have to do this and help yourself." The compassion in her blue eyes told me even more: her genuine concern for a very broken friend. But knowing it came out of love and concern didn't make the stinging comment any more bearable. I sat in silence for a moment.

As I returned to my cubicle, I knew my friend was right, but I wasn't ready. I wasn't ready to explain to a stranger by surrendering and throwing in the towel. The stigma that surrounds seeing a "shrink" was playing with my mind. It would be the mark of another failure on my part, and I couldn't take any more failures. I didn't personally know anyone who'd admitted they needed this type of professional help. People would think I was crazy, and I wanted to fit in every way possible.

A few days after our last talk, I found a small gift-wrapped box and card on my desk. I recognized the handwriting. It was from Penny. In the box was a heart-shaped, pinkish clear crystal. She wrote that crystals have a certain healing power, according to American Indian folklore. She chose this particular one because it contained a single flaw within it. It's believed to ease troubles of the heart and emotions. This was chosen especially for me because she felt I was an unblemished person with a single scar. She prayed that I would find peace from this wound quickly. It would be absorbed into the crystal and remain captured in its inner scar so that I might get on with my life without feeling its torment.

I turned my high-back office chair toward the aisle so that I would be hidden from passing traffic; I felt a tear trickle down my cheek. Closing my eyes, I recalled sitting in this same high-back chair in my cubicle, surrounded with baby shower gifts. Only a year or so before that, I was surrounded with bridal shower gifts. With each flashback, I traced with my finger the photo on my desktop that marked the occasion. Through the years, the acrylic sheet covered them as I slipped each photo under the protective translucent glass, marking a milestone in my life. Each snapshot contained smiling faces of cherished moments, each picture marking another bright dream attained. Those memories were frozen in time, sealed under this plexiglass, a happier, carefree lifetime ago. After tightly grasping the stone for a moment, I placed this crystal on top of my desk and prayed it would soon absorb my misery into its inner scar.

Not too long ago, somewhere in my travels, maybe at church or in the waiting room of the hospital's emergency room, I read a story of an individual looking to purchase a rug. He happened to enter the store from the rear parking lot entrance and walked in, viewing the back of a rug hanging on display. Staring at the back part, he saw only all the knots, crooked, confusing, distorted, and meaningless. Then, as he walked and faced the front of the rug, the pattern, texture, color and combination of the weave revealed a beautiful work of art. Each knot supported the entire design, one after another, until the finished picture was created. The tapestry was now complete.

I realized that Penny was one of the weaves in the pattern of my life. I was fortunate to have her, but, I thought, *Will I survive to see my **finished** tapestry?*

Dark Clouds Become Darker

I would comfort myself at times when I was alone by rocking back and forth and saying, "This is just a dream." I rocked and hummed like a mother would do with her newborn child to help put her baby to sleep. I would do this, repeatedly in threes . . .

"Hum, Mmm; Hum, Mmm; Hum, Mmm."

As I rocked, covered in my old, tattered pink satin-trimmed blanket, I recalled as a young child my mother and father telling me a story during dinner. It was a true story that I would never forget. They told me how my grandfather had left Sicily to come to America after my father was born. He found employment and sent money back to Italy to support his wife and newborn son. After thirteen years of separation, my grandmother and my father arrived in America, where my father met his father for the *first* time since he was a newborn.

If I couldn't see Jacklyn for thirteen *hours*, I would be panic stricken. How my grandfather survived without seeing his only child for thirteen *years* was a sacrifice I couldn't handle. Yet, I thought, coming from such a resilient family, I should be able to handle my current predicament. I needed to get by for only one more day, one more hour, or one more minute.

I wasn't feeling strong enough that day to cope with any emergencies, and I wanted to rock and hum a little longer.

"Hum, Mmm; Hum, Mmm; Hum, Mmm."

As Jacklyn's mother, I needed to correct her problems. Whatever I'd done wrong that caused her to be born this way, I had to fix it and fix it fast. She was growing; the longer it took to find out what was wrong, the longer it could take before she would achieve certain important milestones—saying her first word, sitting up, eating solid food, and taking her first steps. Yes, I yearned for those to happen, so I could shout out with pride at each accomplishment. Then and only then would people know that I hadn't done anything wrong.

Whenever I saw my friends and relatives with their children, I found myself staring into a world that I wanted to be part of—a world I wanted us to belong in. Quietly I watched each step, movement, and visual interaction. A few minutes would go by, but I felt my staring could last forever, drinking in the scenic dance of simple family life. I was imprisoned inside my own imaginary glass box, where

I could see the beautiful world outside, where everything grows and changes. But I stay the same—somehow the sunlight cannot penetrate the container; and, slowly, everything inside my world starts to wither, waste away, and die. Our time was running out.

One day, I returned from work and felt ill to the point that I almost fainted. My first impression was to brush it off. Surely it had to be a result of my stressful work atmosphere and constant worrying about Jacklyn. Maybe I was just dehydrated. I knew my weight had dropped, and I brushed that off, too. Taking off my jacket, I noticed strange red dots on my arms. I went into the bedroom and removed more clothing and noticed tiny red dots on my legs. *Am I having an allergic reaction? What could this be?* Reluctantly, I called to make a doctor's appointment. My family physician had an opening later that night. He examined me and drew blood. I returned home, and, within a brief time, I received a disturbing call from his office.

He ordered me to go directly to the emergency room. He explained that the blood cells known as platelets were lower than normal. My count was only 12,000, when it should have been around 300,000. I could bleed longer if injured or begin to bleed internally or externally for any reason. I could die.

Karl made a few phone calls. Within that brief time, someone, I don't know who, arrived at our home to stay with Jacklyn. Starting from the moment the doctor instructed me to go directly to the emergency room, all my senses started to get fuzzy. Everything became blurry and slowed down to a snail's pace. Even the raindrops hitting the windshield as we drove to the hospital were moving in slow motion. The water was zigzagging across the windshield in jagged patterns that matched my flashbacks of that evening's chain of events.

We arrived at the emergency room, a familiar place for us. I thought, *How ironic—this time, Jacklyn is not with us.* Sitting in the same chair I had used on numerous visits, I mumbled to myself, *What the hell is going on? This can't be happening to me!* After a brief wait, I was called into the office and then sent directly to a nurse's station. As I was being examined, all I kept repeating to the nurse was, "Please hurry. I need to go home and take care of my child. I don't feel sick, so why am I here?"

As I started to get up and leave the ER, Karl took my hand and said, "Sit down. You have to wait here."

I repeated to him over and over again, "I want to go home. I feel fine. I'm not sick. I'm *not* sick!" As I was being rolled down a long hallway on a hospital bed to an elevator, Karl quietly walked alongside the bed, holding my trembling hand. My body was shaking, and I couldn't stop it. As we reached the elevator, he said "Good night." He looked weary. In a soothing voice, he said he would visit tomorrow.

"*No!* Don't come back. It's not necessary," I replied while the doors closed. *Shit! How could I be so mean to him? Why did I say that?* I didn't intend to lash out, but I was so upset that I had become a burden to my already-burdened family. As we reached my floor, the overhead hallway lights flashed past like highway lane dividers leading me in a direction that I didn't want to travel. I was placed in a private room, where the nurse started my medication and checked my vitals.

After one week of testing, my diagnosis was confirmed. In an early-morning visit, my doctor informed me that I had ITP—***I**diopathic **T**hrombocytopenia **P**urpura.*

"What is that?" I whimpered. I couldn't even say my diagnosis! All I could remember from his explanation was that "idiopathic" meant "of unknown cause" and that my blood wasn't clotting as it should.

Later that evening, a priest happened to be making his rounds and asked if I wanted his company and prayers. I said "Yes." After explaining my situation, I asked him, "Why is God doing this to me and my child? I'm a good person. I attend Mass and follow the Commandments, so *why*?" Crying and wanting an answer he could not possibly provide was all I could do now. I was worn out from the day's onslaught; but soon, stillness settled in, surrendering to my fate or maybe the IV's concoction. I felt helpless—*again*—and at the mercy of the medical professionals.

I noticed compassion and genuine concern in the priest's eyes as he was speaking words of encouragement. Not being able to answer my question, he started to pray while leaning over my hospital bed railing. As he bent forward, the ceiling light created an odd yet heavenly glow around him. Before he left my bedside, he placed a small prayer booklet into my hands. He asked me to read it and have faith in God's plan. I did as he asked before falling off to sleep, my teardrops marking each page.

Months passed, and I returned to the hospital numerous times until my doctor advised that surgery to remove what could be a defective spleen was their next recommended step.

The high dosage of steroids kept me up, and then I needed drugs to sleep. Many evenings Karl would urge me to take drugs to sleep after I wanted to start painting the living room at 11:00 p.m. Deep down inside, I knew this medicinal cocktail was making me mentally, physically, and emotionally unbalanced. I knew I had reached the end of my options. I agreed, and the surgery date was scheduled.

Every day before the operation, I wondered repeatedly, *I could die during surgery if my platelets are too low! What if it doesn't cure my disorder?* Tossing and turning with frustration at bedtime only brought on more questions that would spin around in my head: *How much longer can I handle this? Is this the right thing to do? Why is this dark cloud over me and my family? Could God be punishing me for something I did in the past?*

I was scheduled for surgery early Friday morning, and that day, we were hit with a blizzard. I secretly prayed that I would be spared the operation. Bluntly, I was afraid I might die—and then what would happen to Jacklyn? All this fear dissipated as my surgeon entered my hospital room. This stout man stood at the edge of my bed with snowflakes still glistening on his face and clothing, while small chunks of snow slid off his boots and parka. He was not deterred by the snow and prepared to perform my splenectomy. He assured me that my platelet count was high enough, so uncontrolled bleeding should not take place. Karl called as the hospital staff prepared to take me to surgery. He said he would be working from home and would see me later. My reply was simple: "I love you. Goodbye."

Waking up after my surgery, I recall hearing someone state that it appeared to be a healthy spleen!! I mumbled, "What? A healthy spleen? Did I hear that right? What does this mean? Oh, my God, it wasn't bad after all." I was still groggy, but, suddenly, now I was not optimistic. I'd just had major surgery, and there wasn't anything obviously wrong with my spleen!

I couldn't look at my scar. It was ugly: a red-looking rope down the center of my midsection. This keloid scar hurt like hell when anything touched it. My recuperation was spent at home while my mother-in-law and mother helped care for Jacklyn. All lifting was out of the question per doctor's orders, but frankly I didn't need to be reminded because I couldn't even stand up straight. Walking hunched over was the norm for me, as I continued taking various medications but slowly being weaned off the awful steroids.

During my long convalescence, Karl was required to go on a business trip to San Francisco for five days. Since it was the end of my sick leave and I was feeling stronger, we thought it might lift my spirits if I joined him. Distraction from life to a far-off location was so tempting. The notion of possibly seeing the Golden Gate Bridge, cable cars, Lombard Street, and eating Ghirardelli chocolate all excited me. My in-laws offered to care for Jacklyn, so off I went to have this getaway to renew what was left of my spirit. Keeping in mind to follow all my physician's instructions, we flew out to San Francisco, where I planned to rest during the day and have dinner with Karl in the evening.

I was excited as we entered our hotel room. It had simple décor of basically white with beige hues. Our restroom was all white, with a hint of cream-colored tile trim. On the second evening, we retired early because of Karl's early-morning schedule.

I woke up around 4:00 a.m. and felt liquid in my mouth that tasted awful. After a few more times of swallowing this liquid, I went into the restroom and spit out the foul fluid. It was **BLOOD, BRIGHT-RED BLOOD**. I repeatedly spit out more of my blood. I opened my mouth to see large blood blisters on both sides. Now, this previously white serene restroom had red spots splattered over the entire counter and towels. "Shit!" I yelled.

Hearing this, Karl entered the room. Shocked, his eyes widened, eyebrows furrowed, arms reaching out to hold me. He quietly but firmly stated, "Get dressed now; we have to leave and go to the emergency room."

As we entered the hospital's emergency room, I knew exactly what was wrong. I needed to substantially boost my steroids because my platelet count had dropped to a very dangerous level. Surprisingly, there was no one in the waiting room. A blood test was performed and confirmed my fears. My platelet count was a mere 3,000. They wanted to give me a blood transfusion! I insisted they call my New York doctor to prescribe additional prednisone medication. I was fortunate that they did reach him, because getting a blood transfusion in the early days of the AIDS epidemic in San Francisco was a frightening choice. Testing to find clean blood was one of the current topics on the news. The process was new, and very few facilities had it in place.

After popping the extra pills to quickly jack up my platelet count, we returned to the hotel. Karl left for his meeting after changing our return home flight. As in the past, I felt fine, with no indication of this silent killer within me. I then cleaned up the remainder of the blood droplets in the bathroom while blaming myself for Karl missing the rest of his business obligations.

With time to kill before our flight, I considered venturing outside but knew I had to be careful. A simple trolley car ride would be the perfect tourist thing to do before leaving pretty San Francisco. I delicately climbed onto the trolley and cautiously moved around the city for a few hours. It was pleasant to escape even for a fleeting time, to run away from reality, to be someone else who was carefree, not a single problem or worry in the world.

Fisherman's Wharf was bursting with activity. The nearby saltwater and seagulls transported me into another world. I noticed a nearby shop with beautifully displayed oriental items. It drew me in like a bee drawn to a flower's nectar. Behind the counter was a white, silky colorfully embroidered coat. The lady asked if I needed help. Still mesmerized by its splendor, the lady asked me again, saying, "Are you interested in trying on the 'happi coat'?" Hearing that sealed the deal. I walked out with my purchase and hoped it would bring me just that!

Upon exiting at my return trolley stop, the car jolted, and I hit my leg. I went back to my hotel room and started to finish packing in anticipation of our flight. I removed my pants to see this massive bluish-black mark. I had tried to be so careful but again had failed, and failed terribly. By the time Karl returned, my leg turned more toward the color black than blue. Karl looked worried and instructed me to sit while he finished packing. During my return journey, I had plenty of time to reflect. I sat in silence for the entire trip back home. The only words I could speak to him were "I'm sorry."

At home, my doctor determined that I'd had a relapse because my medication had been reduced too quickly. I didn't follow the directions properly. I continued for months to take various drugs while being slowly weaned off the steroids.

I've heard stories and read articles on how the mind can emit chemicals that harm or heal a body. Too much stress and negativity can make you sick. I had to think positive thoughts to stay alive. It felt like I was walking on a tightrope—such a fine line. One foot followed by another, slow and steady, feeling the rope pressing along the bottoms of my sore feet. If I didn't think those good thoughts, I would fall off the tightrope and plunge down into the dark hole—a very dark, deep hole. But if I stayed focused, the path leading to safety was just a few more steps away.

Time passed, and, with the guidance of my new physician, the high dosage of this medication was slowly reduced. Each week as I drove to get blood drawn, my motto became

"Things could be worse," struggling daily to accept and stay positive and think good thoughts. My routine in Jacklyn's care became more systematic, as I knew I had to restore my health, so I could provide the continuous attention she deserved plus remove the extra burden from my husband. I didn't want to be MIA (Missing in Action) at home when it came to her care. I didn't find anything funny anymore, so forcing myself to laugh at a funny movie was a start. Next, just by avoiding talking about Jacklyn during my lunch breaks helped to remove the dull pain in my stomach during the day.

Compelling—even pushing—myself to do something for myself was tough. It was never in my DNA. I forced myself to do something "happy" because it was the healthier mental choice: ultimately, a lesson in retraining my mind to learn how to emit those good chemicals that put you in high spirits. Trying to think positive thoughts and not feel guilty was a tricky task. I discovered ways to minimize my concerns over the fact that I had a seriously sick child. I would place headphones on Jacklyn and let her listen to a Disney book on tape and calculate the amount of time I had to go out and have some so-called fun! It was exhausting.

My weekly blood tests now changed to monthly visits. One month my platelets were at a normal level, and by the next, it had dropped. Visiting Ellen, the nurse specialist, was part of my social activities. Between Jacklyn and I, 75 percent of our socialization was with medical professionals. Ellen would write detailed instructions for me, making sure I didn't screw up my medication. The wrong dosage would really ruin everything to this point. I needed kindness, understanding, and patience. Ellen fulfilled all these needs.

At a routine doctor's appointment, he encouraged me to keep doing whatever I was doing as he continued to wean me off different drugs. I nodded, thanking him for getting me to this point—but what I really wanted to tell him was that it was all a lie. How could I keep up this false happiness? It was impossible!

I had been stable, on fewer pills, but still not myself. I worried that this lie, this falsehood I'd created would catch up to me. Yet, I had to continue to emit those good chemicals in my brain. Otherwise, I might lose my progress.

After a few months, I returned to the doctor's office. It seemed like I was waiting longer than usual for the doctor to see me for this follow-up visit. Finally, he entered, still reading the contents of my folder. I started to sweat, hoping my last blood test didn't show my platelets in another decline. I couldn't go back to all those nasty pills. Inhaling, I took a deep breath. Slowly, he looked up, smiled, and said I was officially in remission. Ecstatic and now with a huge smile on my face, I started shaking his hand and thanked him for healing me. It was a brief feeling of real happiness. Before leaving the office, I stopped at Ellen's desk. She already knew the results and smiled. Thank God—one of my prayers had been answered.

Walk to the Park Swing

I wanted so desperately to have some type of normal routine. I wanted to give Jacklyn happiness and have her experience "childhood" fun. She couldn't talk to me, and right then, I did not need words! Most of the time I can sense; words are created for those children who can use them, but for those who cannot, a mother's love will suffice.

It was a pleasant day, and I planned to take her to a local park. My goal was the playground swing—every child's rite of passage. Overjoyed with my planned trip, I explained "We are going to experience something different today. You are going to fly like a bird." Jacklyn just stared off with no reaction, quiet and non-responsive. I continued to talk while getting her and the chair down the house steps—always the biggest challenge. But, after maneuvering all the steps inside the house to the landing and then several more down the outside of our home, we reached the sidewalk. Reassuring her, I said, "Don't be afraid—we are going to the park to have fun." Then I kissed her cheek and repeatedly caressed her soft, pale face with the palm of my hand. She exhaled; a tiny bubble appeared by her mouth only to quickly disappear as it popped.

Standing at the corner of 7th and Euston Road, I was drawn to the tranquil route: traveling down the quiet streets as opposed to the main road of Nassau Boulevard, with all the hustle and bustle of traffic. Pausing briefly as I eyed both routes, it was clearly a no-brainer!

Off we went down Euston Road to the noisy Boulevard, smelling the fresh-cut grass and listening to the trees rustling in the gentle wind. The huge oaks were full of life, with the birds chirping. Nassau Boulevard had the consistent clatter of cars and trucks whizzing by, accompanied by occasional horns blowing. Jacklyn's eyes widened with delight as she turned in the direction of a passing car whose music was so loud that we could plainly hear it approaching and then leaving our location.

We arrived at Garden City South Park and playground within twenty minutes. Her face lit up when she heard all the children yelling and screaming. The flags on the huge flagpole were flapping in the wind and, in the distance, the echoes of the basketball players dribbling their ball. I looked around and found a corner of the playground that was not being used by other mothers and their children. I rolled her past a smudged, white-chalked walkway to finally stop and remove the straps that held her securely in place. I took a deep breath and then carefully lifted her up onto my lap and slowly backed myself onto the long, narrow rubber seat of the swing. I walked back and forth until we were swinging gently together as one. The squeaking sound from the chains that held the swing were monotonous. In the back of my mind, I considered, *What if the chain doesn't hold us, and we both fall to the ground?* I had to make sure I would cushion her fall. I held her close and at the same time held the chains of the swing as tight as possible. My hands turned red from the pressure put on them. Fingernail marks appeared on my palms. The position was difficult, but I was not going to quit.

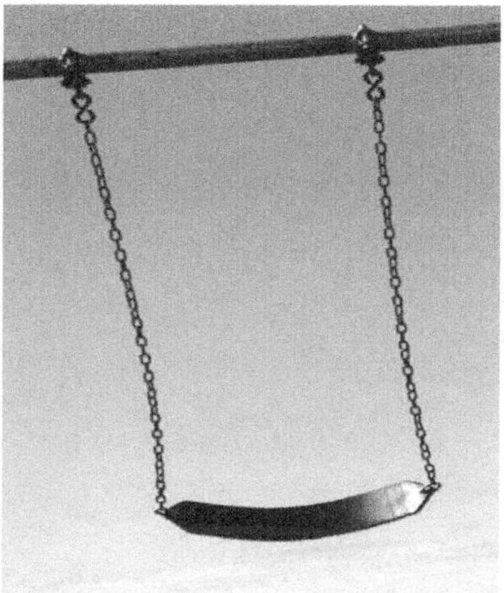

I started to relax, and now it brought me back to my carefree childhood days. An ecstatic feeling rushed over me knowing I was giving Jacklyn what she deserved. I felt so alive, swinging back and forth as the wind brushed our faces. Her hair smelled like newly cut blades of grass with a touch of dewdrops. I was free, like a bird in flight. "Jacklyn, we are flying—wheeeee, wheeeee." On the first few swings, Jacklyn's facial expressions showed her surprise and amazement. She turned her head to me and made a sound that I recognized as cheerful while she raised her fisted right hand to touch her open mouth. How can I explain the communication we had between us when no one else could understand the language?

I yelled out again "wheeeee" with each little swing. "Wheeeee, wheeeee, wheeeee," over and over again, yelling louder and louder with each soft push off the ground. The breeze was gentle, and, as I looked down at her in my arms, I recognized a small smile. She was happy.

She felt it, too—being free as a bird.

"What lies behind you and what lies in front of you pales in comparison to what lies inside of you."

—Ralph Waldo Emerson

Depression and the Deep Hole

To me, depression is like a volcano erupting; except, when it explodes, I end up falling back in and taking a downward plunge deeper and deeper into the darkness.

I was standing alone in a doctor's office, just another one of Jacklyn's appointments. I don't recall the purpose of our visit. Karl couldn't attend with me, so I was listening to the doctor's opinion. I was trying to understand this new, gloomy medical prognosis when all I wanted to hear was how my daughter could be cured. I zoned out and pictured myself clawing and scraping out of a hole. I was suffocating from the dirt burying me, and I was trying to pull myself upward to get a breath of air. My face was barely exposed, and I inhaled, hoping to gain some control. As I took a deep breath, I composed my mind before it raced off in directions that would be of no value and only detrimental to our survival. I was extremely afraid of myself and what I had become. I knew my child didn't realize my incompetence. Her light-brown eyes were focused on the bright lights in the office. I would give anything for her to see me.

As I drove home from this doctor's appointment, Jacklyn had fallen asleep. A small billboard caught my attention, advertising a young couple climbing a mountain. Instantly, I related to the sign. I realized the male hiker carrying the safety rope was Karl, who secured our family; the compass in his hand was the professionals who were attempting to guide us. But, at times, I was standing on the heavy boulder that cracks away and starts plummeting downward, gaining momentum. I would reach out and grasp onto a protruding rock and help anchor myself, until I obtained enough strength and continued the climb to the mountaintop and see the sunrise.

The mental pain and hopelessness that comes with depression was and will always be worse than any physical pain I have experienced. The first time I "clawed and scraped" and made it out of the hole, I found that I was terrified at the thought it could happen again. I didn't want to fall deeper and possibly not have the strength in the next round to make it out alive. Floating in and out of depression can be brought on by many different circumstances. I never knew exactly when or what would make this demon rise.

The Visit

One weekend my relatives from Connecticut planned a visit. We'd grown up together in Brooklyn, and I was looking forward to seeing them again. My aunt and uncle were my godparents, and Valerie and Joseph were more like a sister and brother to me. My cousin Joseph had married, and I was glad that I would be seeing his wife, Annmarie, and their two young sons.

It was 10:00 a.m. as I heard the grandfather clock chime its ten strokes. I expected them to arrive at noon. I became more nervous as the time passed, keeping busy by preparing lunch, rechecking the menu, cleaning, and re-cleaning. Next, half-past-the-hour chimes went off as I finished combing Jacklyn's hair while whispering to her that her cousins would soon be arriving. I made sure I put on Jacklyn's favorite music as I continued to recheck and prepare for our special guests: re-folding and positioning the napkins on the dining room table, fixing the pillows on the living room chairs, checking the bathroom towels and toiletries.

Now, eleven strokes from the grandfather's clock echoed throughout the house. With the anticipation mounting with each passing minute, I thought, *How will they react upon seeing Jacklyn? How would Marc and John, being so young, understand that she cannot communicate with them, see them, or speak? How uncomfortable are these children going to be?* Naturally, I wanted all my guests to have an enjoyable afternoon. As for myself, the demon inside me lay in wait.

The doorbell rang, and Karl glanced at me curiously before opening the door. As my relatives entered the house, I felt smothered, as if the air was sucked out of my lungs and replaced with feelings of sadness and isolation. My cousin Valerie's eyes briefly met mine. I could see the prepared strength she put into her gaze. I felt a lump develop in my throat. A crushing weight was now resting heavily on my chest. A voice in my head screamed, *I'm losing it! What should I do now?* Next, seeing Joe and Annmarie's two healthy and handsome young boys hit me hard—brutally hard.

Before they finished removing their coats, this unexpected emotion forced me to race into the restroom. Karl knocked on the restroom door and asked if I was okay, but I didn't respond. Using a towel, I muffled the sounds that poured out—loud, horrible, echoing sounds that spilled out with a vengeance. My sobbing was still too loud, so I turned on the water at the sink, full force, to suppress and drown out the sounds of my shame. My face was red, my eyes puffy and swollen. I was embarrassed. But the happiness I had for my cousin and his family was genuinely from my heart. My situation was the unforeseen emotional baggage. *Why me? Why her? Why us?* kept repeating in my mind as an image flashed of what *should* have been—our three children playing together. My stomach was in knots as I tried to think what I could talk about!

After a few minutes, I controlled myself and went out to greet my guests. Jacklyn appeared either startled by the new voices or she sensed my emotions. Her thick eyebrows raised, and her eyes widened as her body stiffened. I feared a seizure may be coming on. I kissed her, placed my hand on her cheek and held her hand until she appeared calmer. I continued to keep my cupped hand caressing her left cheek, in fact drawing strength from her as I felt her relaxing.

I placed refreshments on the table, and we started to reminisce about our childhood antics, family vacations, and school days. During their visit, I occasionally glanced over to Marc and John. These two young boys sat quietly with manners far superior then their ages, surely surpassing some adults' behavior that I have unfortunately witnessed. As they observed Jacklyn, their wrinkled brows and innocent faces spoke volumes to me.

I never said a word to anyone about my episodes and wanted to continue to hide my weakness that was quietly eating away at my heart. Lately, it had become something I'd learned to do well.

The Invitation

The envelope had been sitting on the kitchen table. It had been there for two days and I hadn't opened it. From the return address, I knew it was an invitation for a relative's special event—a baby shower. Everyone in my family was attending, so I accepted. I already knew that if I declined, the onslaught of phone calls would have been overwhelming. Speaking to everyone would force me to reveal my current mental state or compel me to lie. After making the commitment, I decided to purchase a gift off the registry. Quickly I entered the baby store, picked out a functional gift, and exited, trying not to view the hundreds of items I could not enjoy that separated my two worlds.

The baby shower day was approaching, and I was anxious, not only for myself but for the parents-to-be. I was a naïve mother-to-be once who looked at life with rose-colored glasses. Now, in fact, seeing anyone—family, friend, or stranger—who was pregnant would immediately invoke a prayer to grant them a healthy baby. As I wrapped the gift, I quietly said "Hail Mary, full of grace, the Lord is with you; blessed are you among women, and blessed is the fruit of your womb, Jesus. Holy Mary, Mother of God, pray for us sinners now and at the hour of our death. Amen." I felt Mary would fully understand why I wanted to pray to her.

Upon entering the beautifully decorated restaurant, a clear bubble surrounded me, and I stared at all the ladies. Everyone was moving in slow motion and speaking, but I did not hear them. A soft crystalline cloud appeared to cover the attendees as I felt totally disconnected from the party. I said another prayer for the mother-to-be as I took my seat and tried to look engaged with the festivities. Should I go up to her and tell her that when her child cries too much, breaks a vase, or climbs on top of the kitchen counter to reach those fresh-baked cookies, to embrace the moment? Should I tell her that, if her child draws on the living room wall, she should be happy and not get angry?

No, no! my inner voice quickly went off. It was so loud that I thought I was shouting "No" for all to hear. As I tried to reconnect with reality, a woman approached me and asked, "How is your daughter Jacklyn?" With my rehearsed response for this type of encounter, I gave a brief update. Her comment was "Oh, she will grow out of it." I nodded, the hair on my arms rose, and I walked away, counting the minutes before the party would be over. Hiding behind a forced smile, I continued to fake my feelings. I'd learned to create this expression from months of practice to cover my pain and fears.

As I watched each gift being opened, I kept a mental tally, focusing on the newborn items that were similar to what Jacklyn had been using and would continue to use. There lay my only connection—the diapers, baby wipes, musical toys, bath chair, baby jars. The other mothers talked about when their children started to eat solid food, stopped using diapers, took their first steps, and said their first word. I had nothing to add to their conversation. I got up and walked away after hearing a mother proudly state that her child recently called her "Momma."

After returning home that night, I dreamt of a gigantic ocean wave hitting and knocking me over. Down I went, gulping in the salty seawater as I struggled to swim upward to the surface. Again, I was hit with another foamy wave, pushing me downward, where the underwater silence was peaceful, calling me to surrender.

The next morning, I woke up still feeling tired and thought that life can change so suddenly. I didn't sleep well, but this time it was different. I was afraid of myself and who I'd become. I guess in some way I will always be broken.

Escape Reality One Day; Slapped in the Face the Next

Some people go to the mall to shop for themselves, buying holiday presents, children's clothing, or household items. I went to the Roosevelt Field Mall to escape my reality. The "escape reality" section is not listed in store directories. Neither Macy's nor Bloomingdale's sells this item. How could anyone wrap that in a gift box?

Karl told me, "Get out of the house for a while, and everything at home will be fine." He promised to handle everything. I don't remember driving there, but one night I found myself walking from store to store, meandering past racks of clothing. I stopped and flipped through sweaters, pants, and then dresses. I gazed at the bright colors and assorted styles and even tried on a few outfits. The seasonal displays at each store window held my attention until another window caught my interest.

I rarely bought anything, yet I received a present each time I went to the beautifully decorated stores. "Attention customers: This store will be closing in fifteen minutes," a loud voice projected. Many last-minute shoppers headed to the cashier as I headed out the door. The fresh air and stillness of the parking lot rejuvenated me, and I felt a renewal of some kind as I slowly strolled along the wet pavement to my car. I was alone in my own world.

The car was running, and my favorite radio station was blasting. The lights attached to the huge parking light poles cast a sparkle on the mist that overshadowed the lot. It was a gloomy vision—complete stillness and total quiet except for the occasional passing car off in the distance. Now, my guilt took me to another level. *I'm not fit to be a mother!* I was out having fun while my child was home fighting for another day. Would I regret these frivolous few hours if she is gone tomorrow?

As I pulled into the driveway, I noticed that the bedroom lights were out. I quietly walked into her room. Holding my breath, I slowly approached her bed. As I bent over, I exhaled—she was alive. She was awake. Her eyes were wide open; she was listening to every sound. Did she know I hadn't been home? Was she waiting, or did I wake her when I opened the front door? "I'm sorry," I whispered. Taking my fingertips, I gently traced the top of her eyebrows and continued toward her hairline. I repeated this with soft strokes until her eyes started to close. Then tucking her teddy bear blanket around her while kissing her cheek, I said, "I love you. Good night."

One Sunday morning, Karl was heading out to do some errands and said he would be gone for most of the day. I nodded and then placed Jacklyn on the changing table to give her a fresh diaper. While watching me, he reached out and squeezed my hand until I gave him my full attention. I guess my mental struggles were clearly apparent to him. Then, looking into my eyes, he said that I "could step up to the plate or pack it in." It was my choice.

It was straightforward and simply said, without need for discussion or explanation. He said it out loud, and I knew exactly what he meant. Those unspoken thoughts had now been put into words. I felt the power of his statement, and his cutting words were sharper than a knife. It was my new reality, slapping me in the face—the stinging, hard, cold truth. I thought I had a secret that was locked up in the corner of my mind. No one else could see the truth, subconscious, hidden from sight. But he saw me clearly. I couldn't hide it from him—my thoughts of taking back the tormented, innocent life I created, along with my tortured one.

As I looked down at Jacklyn, I repeated his words in a whisper, "Step up to the plate or pack it in; step up to the plate or pack it in; step up to the plate or pack it in."

Counselor at Work

Weeks after my return to work, a co-worker called me into his office. He wanted to give me some advice. He suggested that I sign up for counseling that was sanctioned by the company. He was wise enough or had some experience that this would not only help me mentally, but possibly stop the harassment by management. At this point, waging two wars was exhausting, and I needed help. I was feeling run-down, mentally, physically, and emotionally.

I didn't know what to expect from a company counselor. Nevertheless, I signed up and met him in his office the next day. He was a jovial, middle-aged man. We talked and scheduled routine meetings. Each week we discussed different topics, from world news to how I would deal with the next medical evaluation. He had a few goals for me, but one short-term one was to go out to dinner with my husband and leave Jacklyn at home in the care of a sitter. This task seemed simple to most, but our routine meetings quickly went from weeks to months without this having been accomplished. I pondered why I had not progressed to the point of going out to dinner. Maybe I was too broken, or maybe his skills were limited and could not get me there sooner. I felt it was a combination of both scenarios.

One year later, I finally felt strong enough to arrange a night out for dinner at a local restaurant. This was different from going to a mall and escaping *my* world. I was taking the next step. It was a form of acceptance of our current state of affairs. I still felt at fault for Jacklyn's condition and that I didn't deserve this night out. It brought back memories of how our life was before the tragic turn. I was stuck in a time warp right before her first seizure.

Roseann, my niece, arrived at our home. Sensing my distress, she had a somber expression and avoided eye contact with me. We kissed each other's cheek, and she sat on the couch after greeting Karl. She was a mother of Jennie, Michael and Laura—three healthy, beautiful children. Her familiarity with my baby's routine gave me some solace.

I put on a Disney DVD and hoped Jacklyn would enjoy hearing the cute voices in the movie. Karl had already given her physical therapy and postural drainage to keep her lungs clear. I started to get dressed but felt sick to my stomach. I could not believe I was going out to have "fun" and leaving Jacklyn. *What kind of mother am I?* I knew from all my counseling sessions that this was a step I needed to take. But it still felt wrong. Karl deserved better, so I finished getting dressed for our dinner date.

We drove a short distance and parked in the restaurant lot adjacent to a Long Island Railroad crossing. I started to break out in a cold sweat as we walked up the pathway to the restaurant. With a slight smile, Karl gallantly held the front door open for me.

We ordered dinner and tried to make small talk. I sensed he was trying hard not to discuss anything remotely related to our child's future. He appeared uncomfortable but did a noble job of keeping our date as pleasant as he could under the circumstances. I thought to myself that he had to be hurting, too, but concealed it well for the sake of our marriage and for my mental survival. This was a big step for me, and he knew it!

I floated in and out of listening to him discuss current world news as if I had the television remote in my hand: pressing the mute button ON and then after some time pressing it OFF. I had a glass of wine to help me relax, but it didn't work. I still felt sick to my stomach but didn't tell Karl. Why should I ruin the night for him, too? He had worked so hard to keep Jacklyn and myself safe. When we were dating, he always enjoyed going out to have a pleasant dinner. He should at least be able to receive this simple pleasure. Now, those memories of when we started dating and planning for our future seemed like a lifetime ago.

Karl asked for the check, and I wanted some fresh air, so I told him I would meet him at our car. Quickly putting on my coat, I left the building. Tears started rolling down from my eyes. I wanted to rid my head of the torment, but I didn't know how to achieve this freedom. Mental pain is much worse than physical pain. There is no comparison.

It was a foggy night, and instead of walking to the car, I started to walk to the railroad crossing gate that had just come down. The warning bells rang while lights flashed. I could see off in the distance the dim light of a train approaching. I stood next to the tracks as the train came closer. The fog was getting thicker, and a soft mist was in the air, gently hitting my face. It felt like a veil made of tiny teardrops. I thought that so many people end their mental pain this way. It would be quick. I would be free. I'm not afraid to die, but afraid to live. The train was a quarter-mile away as I swayed back and forth. My eyes filled with tears.

Karl's comment days ago—"Step up to the plate or pack it in; step up to the plate or pack it in"—bounced around in my head.

A blurry image of Jacklyn sitting alone flashed before me. Sitting alone!! Alone and unprotected!! With that vision, I slowly turned and walked toward our car. I could feel the wind from the passing train whirling at my back. My long black coat flapped outstretched from the enormous gust that surrounded me.

Picturing Jacklyn without a mother to defend and take care of her wasn't an option. As I sat in the car, I knew Karl needed and deserved as much help as I could provide, no matter what I could handle at any given time. This precious child had made us a team. I forced a smile as I turned to Karl and asked, "Did you enjoy your dinner?" His positive response was weak but clear.

In a way that night, Jacklyn saved *me*!

Therapist Calls at Home

I confided in my co-worker Penny whenever possible during lunch. She realized I needed a more-trained professional therapist. But, after-work appointments seemed excessive and time consuming. I didn't have extra time to spare. I never wanted to seek any outside help. The one-on-one basis made me feel uncomfortable. Bottom line, I knew they couldn't give me what I desperately sought. So, why should I bother? It was pointless to complain to a stranger. Why would they care? I was in a dismal position, torn between a friend's advice and denial that it would help me.

At times, I found myself awkwardly avoiding Penny while navigating our office cubicle maze. I couldn't face her because I knew she was right. I had the same feeling I'd experienced when I was a schoolgirl and entered the classroom, facing the teacher without my completed homework. I had not done what was asked of me.

Day after day, that feeling lingered until it broke me. I made the appointment. Most visits were uneventful, but there were times that I walked a fine line, almost falling back deeper into the dark hole. The reoccurring topic centered on the fact that since I carried Jacklyn, I must have done something to cause her disability. This tormenting question constantly circled in my mind. It must have been the wine I drank before I found out I was pregnant. Maybe, it was the tuna fish I had eaten at lunchtime when I went out with the girls, or the paint I inhaled as I passed by the new nursery room Karl was painting. Did I play with some harmful chemicals when I was a child? Could it be a combination of all those events? What did I do? What?

It was a cold Friday night at dinnertime, and Karl had gone away on a business trip. It was a short trip, but it was the first time I was totally alone to handle all the responsibilities. Karl's recent comment on how I could "step up to the plate or pack it in" echoed in my mind. He saw how damaged I had become. I could try to hide it from myself but not from him. Karl left me alone that night, and I thought how easy it would be to turn the oven on and just open the door, allowing the gas vapor to fill the house so we would be at peace together. Two simple steps: turn a knob, open the door. It would be done, and we would both escape this prison.

But no, deep down, a force erupted within me, and I wanted to step up to the plate and hit a home run: a home run to win the game and make the team proud. Sitting at the kitchen table, I reread "Footprints in the Sand" as I rocked back and forth and thought, *Things could be worse.* Oh, yes, it could be so much worse. I continued rocking back and forth while reminiscing when I was a child and my parents rocked me in their protective arms until I fell asleep.

The 10" x 8" white lined paper on the kitchen counter outlined in detail Jacklyn's schedule. During the evening, I followed, checking off each task.

1. Physical therapy—check.
2. Medication—check.
3. Dinner of pureed chicken and rice—check.
4. Thickened liquids—check.
5. Tactile play time—check.

I picked up the tiny doll that had the soft curls, recalling the day I bought it as a Christmas present. I remembered that moment—how it satisfied my need and would give Jacklyn enjoyment, too. It gave me peace then, and it still magically did now. Taking the soft curls from the doll I brushed it against Jacklyn's pale white cheeks and along her thin arms. "Tickle, tickle" I whispered as I held her close. She opened her mouth, and her eyes widened while she turned her head toward me. "Tickle, tickle, tickle," I said as I kissed her cheek. I wiped the drool away from her face as she turned toward the doll, while I fantasized she was saying "Momma" instead of the toy. I continued to daydream, as I gently pressed the button over and over again, hoping that someday I could hear that word.

It was about one hour later that the phone rang. It turned out to be Sharon, my new therapist. She asked, "What did you have for dinner? What did you give Jacklyn for dinner? Did she eat well? Was Jacklyn already sleeping? How are you handling this night without Karl?" The more questions she asked, the more it became apparent. A cold chill ran through my body, giving me the shakes.

As soon as my quivering stopped, I responded softly, "Thank you, Sharon. I understand the main reason for you to get in touch with me tonight."

She seemed surprised by my frankness, with "Oh, you do!" I assured Sharon we both were fine.

It was getting late, so I tucked Jacklyn into bed, and, with the help of her music box, she was asleep within minutes. I stood over her, softly crying and admiring the beautiful baby I'd brought into this world. How I created her and how I hated the evil thoughts that considered taking her away. I detested the devil that hid in the corner of my mind and wished somehow to eradicate the demon.

Before long, I turned off my bedroom light and started to doze off, realizing, *Sometimes you need more than one rope to climb up out of a dark hole.* Tonight, I had three. Yes, three. One, a new therapist, two, my soul mate, and the third did not need a rope. This is because He carried me.

Lake George Vacation

Jacklyn was going to be two years old, and we decided to take a family summer vacation upstate. Lake George was the destination, and my in-laws would join us. Their offer gave me the incentive. I couldn't pass up having Grandma and Grandpa babysit a few nights so I could have time with my husband. It could be 120 minutes or 60 minutes or even 20—I valued every minute I could escape. I thought of how my yesterday was spent and all my days before that, too.

I would wake up each morning and slowly walk over to the crib to see if Jacklyn was alive. If she wasn't, I fantasized how I would pick her up, kiss her, and, while holding her in my arms, say, "You are my beautiful child and I am sorry, oh so sorry. You deserved better, and I failed as your protector. I tried to do my very best and hope you forgive me." I wouldn't call anyone because then they might take her away from me. I would wait for Karl to come home because he would know what I should do.

Each morning while the sun was sending rays that ricocheted around her scalloped bedroom window shades, I gently released the guardrails. I would gradually bend over the crib railing to get close to her face. Slowly peeling back the comforter, I was able to feel her warmth and smell the sweetness of baby shampoo. I saw the slow up-and-down movement of her tiny chest and upper body. With relief, exhaling through my tight lips, I let out a deep, prolonged release of air.

God had given Jacklyn to me for another day, and I thanked Him while I asked that He always watch over her. My daily routine continued with physical therapy, medication, and carefully feeding her meals, avoiding choking or aspiration.

Mealtimes were a slow process. I loved holding her close, letting her feel my presence even though my back, shoulder, and leg ached. I would place each spoonful of food into her mouth and gently press down on her tongue, releasing it. I made sure that all liquids were thickened before pouring each mouthful. As I watched her consume her meal, I couldn't tell if she enjoyed the different textures and tastes except for her occasional wide-eyed expressions. After every fifteen minutes, I would give her circular rubs on her back to get those tiny burps. I cheered her on as I whispered, "Come on sweetie—give Momma a burp." Most of the time, a burp or hiccup would be followed by a slight smile—the cutest of smiles, showing me she was content. Those little smiles gave me peace, a welcome serenity that erased for a few moments some of my pain because I knew she was happy. Next, depending on the day, I would give her a warm bath with the help of a special supportive bath chair,

The physical part was only a fraction compared to the mental drain. My days would always include an attempt to visually connect. At times, I would use a light, mimicking how the doctor would exam her vision. I would stare into her eyes, wishing miraculously to get back a meaningful reaction; but, instead, I would be met with emptiness.

The realization that I must do this and anticipate all her needs *forever* alarmed me. I could not get sick. A few days might be fine, but I couldn't afford to become ill for a lengthy period. To make matters worse, what would happen if Karl got sick, too? I wanted a vacation to escape, even for a few hours.

Call it respite or whatever, but this time alone, so preciously needed for me to be with my husband and free of worry, was worth its weight in gold. Knowing that she would be in safe, trusted hands allowed that little switch in my head to click "off." This knob had been turned "on" for so many hours, minutes, and days that, when it was given the opportunity to switch "off," the peace that would overtake my entire body was heavenly.

The night that our plans were finalized, I dreamt a childhood fantasy—back to the make-believe land where princes and princesses lived, and the fairytale always had a good ending. The noble prince killed the evil dragon, so they would live happily ever after. Indeed, I had the noble prince, but the dragon still lived.

I sat in the seat next to Jacklyn as we started our car journey upstate. I wanted to be close if any problem arose. The concern I felt going on such a long drive was less of an issue than I expected because Jacklyn slept most of the way. It was getting dark, and an uneasy feeling came over me as we entered the nearly filled parking lot of the hotel. It was a two-story structure. The stairs going to the second floor looked like they would be a grueling climb for us with Jacklyn's chair. I felt a bit light-headed and struggled to keep calm until Karl returned to the car, confirming our room would be on the first level, as promised.

As I unpacked our clothing and then changed her diaper, the small hotel room started to fill with the comforts of home. I took out my packing list to make sure I hadn't missed something. Baby food—check. Thickening power for liquids—check. Medication—check. Doctor contact numbers—check. Diapers and wipes—check. Bibs and towels—check. Homemade frozen pureed meals—check. Physical therapy ball—check. Brace—check. Bath chair—check. Music box—check. Plenty of changes of clothing—check.

After such a long ride, Karl wanted to give her physical therapy to help keep her lungs clear. Our home therapists called it "cupping and clapping." To me it was such a funny name but appropriate. I watched as Karl placed her in front of him and gently patted her upper chest; then, after a few minutes, he patted each of her sides. I wondered what would happen when she grew.

Caught daydreaming, Karl yelled out to me, "Lucille, a little help here." I snapped out of it and helped position her face down over the large rubber ball, quickly tucking a small, soft towel under her face. We both lightly pounded and then rubbed her upper back as she was draped head down over the ball. Warm admiration traveled over me in waves as I looked at Karl and how we worked together as a team. Jacklyn appeared to be enjoying her physical therapy by making little sounds. They were happy grunts. There have been times the sounds she expressed and her facial cues showed me her displeasure. It was my signal that the towel I'd placed under her face was soaked with drool.

Ten or fifteen minutes passed, and we were ready to venture out and explore. At this point, I let out a sigh of relief, thinking that this might all work out just fine. The butterflies in my stomach were disappearing, and I tried to let go of the haunting feelings that I didn't deserve any enjoyment while there were so many unresolved issues.

It was close to dinnertime, so we all decided on a nearby German restaurant. The décor was dark and rustic, with wood tables. My mother-in-law was seated at my right, and Jacklyn was in her special chair on my left. Karl and his dad were seated across from us. It was not crowded, and we enjoyed a nice dinner of sauerbraten and bratwurst. At this point, Jacklyn had to be part of our dinner, so I fed her a jar of baby applesauce. I tried to continue and control my nervousness of being so far away from the hospitals we frequented. Perhaps, as my body calmed and the wine warmed me, this vacation could turn out to be a very pleasant experience that, hopefully, we could look forward to again next year.

We had coffee, and then the check was placed on the table. Karl and his dad looked at the check and appeared puzzled. I picked it up and noticed there was an extra charge on it that we all did not understand. I asked the waitress, "What was the additional fee?"

She told me that, while pointing to Jacklyn, "She didn't eat but took up a seat in the restaurant, so there was a charge for that space."

I said, turning to my mother-in-law, "Did I hear her correctly?" I almost lost my composure at the dinner table and instead quickly dashed into the nearby restroom. I yelled, "How could this waitress be so insensitive? What kind of rules do restaurants follow? Is this their company policy for the handicapped? No one could be that callous! What the hell is going on here?" It was clearly apparent that Jacklyn could not eat their food. I held back the tears as my mother-in-law entered the restroom to see how I was coping. I felt such outrage. Angry, fuming, irate, livid—I was going to explode. I pounded the wall with my fists as tears rolled down my cheeks. Thank God, no other patrons were in the restroom to see me rant. What the hell was the waitress thinking—or, worse yet—been instructed to do?

I don't know what was greater—the fury I felt over this action, or the deep pain I felt knowing Jacklyn would be unprotected and taken advantage of by people like this. She was helpless, and there would be other injustices that follow. I had to protect her—become her eyes, ears, and voice forever. It was a slap in the face, a wake-up call that I must become a soldier in a crusade against discrimination in a war I did not want. The pleasant experience I'd hoped for today died at dinnertime.

United Cerebral Palsy Association of Nassau

Since Jacklyn could not attend a traditional school, we had to make plans for the alternative. Our research found that United Cerebral Palsy of Nassau Children's Learning Center would be the most appropriate facility and close to home. As Karl and I sat outside our local school's planning board's office, waiting to be called into the room, I shuddered to think what would happen if they didn't approve our petition.

The door opened, and a man said, "Mr. and Mrs. Messina, please come in." My hand trembled as I shook hands with the parent advocate, special education teacher, and special education chairperson. Fortunately, all went well, and, at age three, an Individual Education Plan (IEP) would be authorized in our school district.

Upon leaving, a bit more relaxed with our success, I looked at the children's drawings and mementos that were proudly displayed on the hallway walls. Somehow, I was drawn to each handmade artwork like a moth attracted to bright light. As I examined each illustration, my stomach started to twinge. Pictures flashed in my mind of all the "should have been" moments. Instead, now I felt cheated by the ironic turn of events. I walked fast to exit the building and quickly removed myself from a place that should have been her school.

Jacklyn continued to have physical therapy at home, and her therapist recommended she be fitted for leg braces. She explained that these molded-plastic foot braces would be beneficial in keeping her calf muscles from contracting. Part of me didn't want this for her, but, like the upcoming admission to UCPN, it was in her best interest. I went through the motions in preparation for these future changes, constantly reminding myself it was the only option we had for now.

A casting and fitting were done by a local orthopedic provider. Upon receiving these small leg supports, I rushed out and purchased a pair of sneakers with Velcro that were oversized, so the braces would slip in easily. Simple satin slippers with elastic trim would work for the very few times I placed her in a dress. This orthotic was easy to use but still upsetting for me to place her little legs in them.

When we attended Sunday Mass, I would find myself staring at other little girls' shoes and thought how lucky those parents were to buy a pair of fancy shoes and pretty dresses. As I watched this one family, their two little girls ran and twirled round and round. Jacklyn became alert upon hearing the children's voices and seemed pleased as she turned in their direction. The younger girl had a pair of Mary Jane–style shoes, sparkly with little bows. The older sister had a little chunky heel with a thin strap. As I watched them, I felt as different as Jacklyn, the odd person out! Peeking out from the corner of my eye so they wouldn't notice me staring, I absorbed every whirl and spin to memorize the beauty of a little girl's youthful prance. My eyes hurt from the strain but continued to be engrossed with their every turn.

My lips recited the "Hail Mary," and I quietly prayed for a miracle as Mass ended. I imagined Jacklyn twirling and dancing until I noticed that her leg-brace strap had opened and was dangling near the footing of her wheelchair. Kneeling by her chair, I repositioned and fastened it correctly. Staring at the white strap that was now in my hand, the dancing image slowly vanished as the girly giggles faded away.

The first day of school was approaching, and I could feel the excitement in the air around our neighborhood. As I was picking up some needed items at our local drugstore, I found myself in line with other mothers who were purchasing school supplies. Their children were asking for cute accessories to make their first school day more fun. "Mommy please, oh please, buy this for me." I tried to relate to these mothers, but it was a poor association. We were so strikingly different. I couldn't link myself because I was that single piece of chain that had a gap big enough to slip the other closed link through the space and fall apart. I was barely holding on, and, depending on what direction it moved, it could easily break away from the rest of the links.

As I prepared myself, it was not going to be as I dreamed. My little girl would not be posing on her first day of school in her pretty new outfit, new lunchbox, backpack filled with her notebook, pencils, and crayons. No, I would not videotape her walking onto the school bus and watch her wave goodbye. That image disappeared as did another piece of my heart.

The school bus arrived, and I assisted the aide in getting the wheelchair onto the bus. I kissed Jacklyn and walked to the curb as the doors closed. As the bus pulled away, I ran along the side of it waving, even though I knew she couldn't see me. I noticed her little face turning in the direction of my voice. Nearly on my toes, I strained to see her through the back window as the bus turned down the block. I started running, following the slow-moving yellow bus as I waved and yelled, "Jacklyn, have a good day."

Soon it turned onto the main road of Nassau Boulevard, where I stopped, went back home, and jumped in my car. Trying not to speed, I got onto the Southern State Parkway and headed to the United Cerebral Palsy Center in Roosevelt. While driving by the few exits, all I could imagine was how my child was feeling being surrounded by strange voices and sensing a strange place. Maybe she was thinking I had abandoned her, afraid, alone, and not able to tell anyone.

We had pre-planned my visit for her first day of class. Entering the complex, I spotted a visitors-only parking spot and barely had the car's gears locked in Park before I jumped out and headed for the front door. I quickly signed in to the office and was taken to Jacklyn's room, passing many different-sized wheelchairs and modified tricycles neatly parked outside each classroom.

As I entered the classroom, a tall, slender young man welcomed me. "Hello, my name is Kurt, and I'm Jacklyn's teacher." He was about my age, had dark, shaggy hair and kind eyes, and was soft spoken. Interrupted by an aide, Kurt directed his attention to her and one of his students. I examined the room while still standing in the doorway entrance. The children in his class had verbalization issues among other problems, and most were in molded tumble forms chairs that had straps for support. Unrecognizable words echoed within the bright room that was filled with various adaptive equipment and floor mats. I was overwhelmed by my own ignorance. How naïve of me! I would rarely see a special child at the mall, so seeing so many children with twisted bodies in one room was devastating. How could I have prepared for this? Even going to the hospital on so many occasions with Jacklyn could not come close to this magnitude for me. Each child had a little person locked inside, each with a different story: from trauma at birth to car accident casualty—any situation was distressing to me. Yet, knowing a child's abilities before a vehicle accident would put a different level of anguish and guilt on a family. Somehow, I could feel in the pit of my stomach the agony they must be enduring.

As I quietly viewed the children in the classroom, I could see beyond their outer shell into the person inside. Sometimes their eyes communicated, or a gesture, nod, even a slight sound in their own way was reaching out, communicating from their world to mine as long as I allowed them in. A little girl was being fed by an aide, and after each spoonful of pureed fruit, her eyes glanced down to the opened jar as if to say, "I'm ready for another." I could sense that here in this classroom, words were not needed to get a passing grade.

Kurt turned to me and started to explain that Jacklyn's day would start by welcoming her. He continued by stating they "would provide a variety of stimulation to include visual, auditory, vestibular, tactile, and olfactory." Each child was treated like they understood, because one does not assume they did not. Upon hearing this, I had an instant connection because I felt the same way. I had a sense that, in this classroom, everyone spoke the same language—understanding, commitment, respect, dedication, and, most of all, love. Kurt's gentle manner and desire to make sure each child was comfortable assured me this experience would make a wonderful fit for Jacklyn and for me.

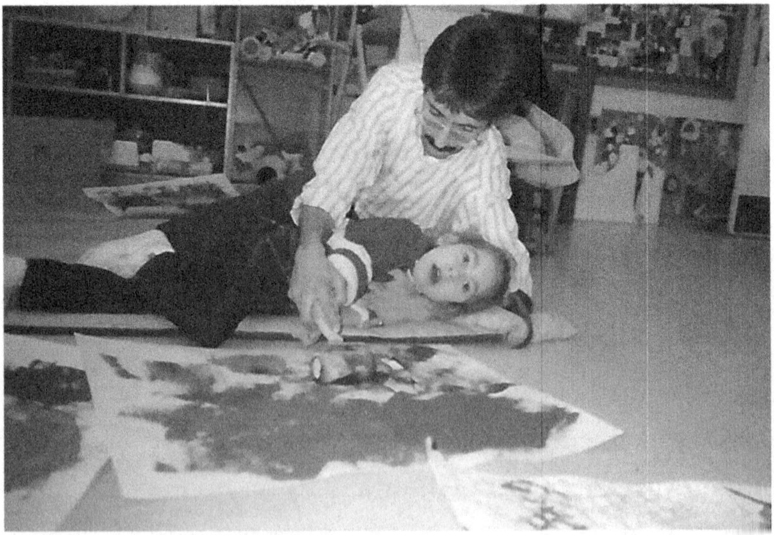

A few months passed, and one day I needed to drop off a change of clothing to her classroom. In my haste, I forgot earlier to pack an emergency outfit. I had gotten accustomed to the routine, but that morning Jacklyn was taking her time eating breakfast. Slow in swallowing each mouthful, she was more interested in focusing on all the noises around her rather than enjoying her meal.

As I entered the classroom to hand the items to an aide, I noticed that one of Jacklyn's classmates was missing. He usually was seated next to Jacklyn and almost always had an infectious grin. While pointing to the empty spot, I said with a smirk, "Is he playing hooky today?"

The aide took me aside and whispered, "He passed away over the weekend." Staring into her now-watery eyes, my body started shaking. I tried to stop shaking, tried to compose myself while processing this news. I thought, *God, I guess you needed another angel.* The aide slowly walked away while wiping a fallen tear off her cheek.

Oh, Lord—it could have been my daughter. I thought about the boy's parents and at the same time pictured myself in their shoes. I kissed Jacklyn, told her "I'll see you later, sweetie," and left the room. Dabbing tears from my eyes, I wondered if the other children noticed that he was missing.

My car was parked at the end of the lot. As I walked, the fresh cool air hitting my face revived me. I noticed most of the trees had lost their leaves by now, but I saw one yellow—almost golden colored—leaf slowly breaking away from the top branch and making its way to join the others. Then, another leaf, more green than yellow, also floating in this descending plunge. They both floated to the left, and then a gust of wind took them to the right. As they gently floated, another gust pushed them upward toward the top of the tree again, only to re-start their downward plunge when the wind calmed down. The yellow-golden one hit the ground. Just like this young boy, who'd lost his battle to stay afloat, so did this golden leaf.

Reaching my vehicle, I noticed the other, greener leaf had fallen and was stuck within a small branch cluster. The super-thin twigs, almost like fingers interlocking like a hand, kept this single leaf from hitting the ground. How appropriate. It was a sign, as I compared my child's struggle to stay afloat—to land on another branch and stay there a little bit longer. Jacklyn was being held high by the supporting thin twigs of Mother Nature, secured until another gust of wind comes along. Or until another medical emergency changes her future. Driving home, all I could think about was, *It could have been Jacklyn—it could have been my child.*

Months passed, and a Family Day Picnic was planned at the end of Jacklyn's first year. It was held outside, and the day was perfect. Not too sunny or hot—just the right amount of cloud cover, gentle breeze, and mild temperature for the students and their families. The children were excited as they were moved out of the classrooms onto the grass. Different stations were set up to play beanbag toss, and they had a face-painting booth, too. I realized that the work involved to plan such an event by the staff was enormous.

It was getting near closing time, and I rolled Jacklyn over to get her face painted. The young girl volunteer gently painted a purple heart on each of her cheeks. She placed a little orange dot on her chin and at each mouth corner, finishing up with orange lines above her eyebrows. Upon completion, I noticed something. Jacklyn's face was remarkably different. She had the sweetest smile! I could feel and see her happiness. After taking a photo with her teacher Kurt, I left that day contented and blessed to have witnessed Jacklyn's very own expression of joy—a freeze-frame moment to lean on when I need to be in a happy place.

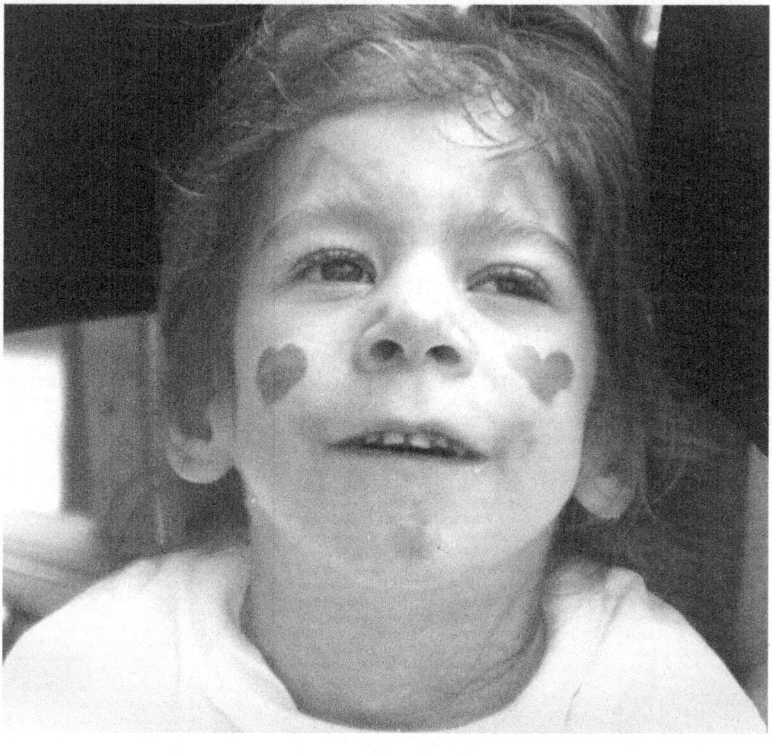

The three years spent at UCPN turned out to be wonderful for Jacklyn and us as a family. My prior frustration would be best explained as if I had been trying to put a square peg into a round hole. It was never going to work. The isolation I felt before diminished as Karl and I found a place to fit in as parents. We all were accepted and included in the United Cerebral Palsy family. They guided and advised us regarding her wheelchair, back brace, leg braces, and a multitude of other medical and personal issues we encountered. Karl even found the time to join the FACE group. It was run by Kurt and was an acronym for the Father and Child Experience. They went camping, boating, pumpkin picking, and to baseball games together. Just like any other mother fondly watching her child and husband bonding and doing day trips, I, too, got to feel that joy.

A classroom notebook was used to communicate from teacher to parent. This little notebook was a lifeline of precious messages that any parent of a non-verbal child would treasure. I felt a sense of peace and shed some of my guilt for not being with her every minute whenever I read the high points of the day so thoughtfully scribed onto a simple piece of paper.

Medicaid

Time passed, and Jacklyn had had this damn scoliosis brace for a few years. She couldn't talk and explain to me how she feels, neither could she move to position her body. She had grown, and I found that each new brace became bigger and more difficult to use. Now, I needed help! I couldn't do it alone. It's morning, and I must get her dressed for the day.

"Mom," I called out, while quietly I was thinking that I'm so thankful that she slept over to provide a helping hand. Yet, why didn't I say, "Thank you" more often to her and others? I wondered at times, what had happened to me. Had I become tired of saying "Thank you," or had I become cold to feelings? I thought I had put up a wall to protect myself and lost the person I once was. I wondered, *am I still in denial?* Because if so, it was the greatest of all my defenses. As I looked at my mother's face, I noticed her eyes. They appeared to be little slits, barely open, a bit red and watery. I could see my face in hers. She stood next to me, waiting for instructions.

I lifted Jacklyn; her eyes and mouth were wide open. I'd noticed the extra weight gain. She started to stiffen her body. Before I could safely finish placing her on the changing table, I felt a sharp twinge in my lower back that warned me to be extremely careful, trying to recall the instructions a nurse had given me during one of her hospital visits. I just couldn't afford to hurt myself. I told Jacklyn, "I'm sorry, but I have to do this."

I called out, "Mom, slide the back part of the brace a little more upward while I reposition Jacklyn onto it." I explained, "She is still too low on the back part." I felt that it was only a matter of time before I would not be able to use the changing table any more. I needed more space. Finally, I aligned the top strap. Immediately I heard a low moan, and her face grimaced. "Shit—it's pinching her skin, and the tee shirt is caught on the metal loop." I continued to adjust the two pieces, so they would meet.

"Okay, sweetie, now I can put you into your chair." I took a deep breath and leaned against the wall for a few seconds. I was sweating and feeling like I needed another shower. Oh, my God: Jacklyn was grunting and turning her head from side to side. Something was wrong! Her face was turning red. I muttered to myself, *What's wrong with me? I did it again.* Without delay, I loosened the bottom strap, so she could breathe easier. I tried not to mentally beat myself up. I'd made a mistake, but everything was fine now. I had to be more careful.

Before I put her sweater on over the brace, I rubbed lotion under her arm to help protect any skin that might rub against the plastic. Then, I continued to massage some lotion onto her thin arms. They were clearly absent of any muscle mass, limp and baby soft. I thought she was enjoying the "spa" treatment as I continued to rub more lotion. Oh, how I wished she could hug me, wave to me, hold a toy! Despite that, I rubbed them as Aladdin would rub his magic lamp to get three wishes from the genie. I thought, *Lord, please. Can just one of my wishes come true?* The feel of the cream in my hands was cool and soothing. The smell of the baby lotion traveled upward, filling my senses and triggering images back in time to my first experience with the brace when she was just a few years old.

First Fitting

Entering the orthopedic provider's office for the first time, I stared at these vest-style, rigid-plastic shell braces and shuddered, realizing my daughter, who was not even four years old, was there for her initial casting. They lined the outer wall and looked terribly uncomfortable. Each vest varied in size and was labeled with other children's names: Cindy, Matt, Julie, and Tommy. Matt's brace was the larger one, with a few pen marks across the top, and Julie was the next in size, with puppy dog stickers all over the front. It crossed my mind numerous times not to use the brace; but, what happens in six months or a year, when it becomes too late, and her spine is left curved and permanently twisted?

Weeks passed, and her first scoliosis brace was finished. Now Jacklyn has leg braces *and* a scoliosis jacket. I hated the thought that now she had to wear both daily. I detested, loathed, despised that it had come to this! This was not a "first time" milestone I wanted to remember.

Every morning, I would glare at them leaning against the wall of her bedroom: rigid and strong, defying me, almost challenging me not to use them. The temptation was compelling. Taking a deep breath, I snatched them up, placing these supports onto her changing table. Bearing in mind my prior instructions, I positioned her shoulders just above the top rear section of the jacket. "I'm sorry, Jacklyn. This is truly hurting me more," I said while kissing her chest. Next, I rubbed some baby lotion on her upper body, put her tee shirt on, and then lowered the top piece to encase her full torso. Making sure I didn't pitch her skin, I secured the Velcro straps that connected the two pieces of molded plastic. The straps had to be tightened but not too tight. I could only imagine the discomfort—being wrapped in a hard plastic jacket every day to keep my body straight.

The warmth of summertime was awful. I didn't look forward to that season, like most families did. Her cotton tee shirt would always be necessary to wear, no matter how high the temperature. The heaviness of the air and her perspiration-soaked shirts would be a constant reminder of her distress. I felt helpless and like a monster for torturing my child. I would watch the other children running, playing—brace-free—as my insides ached. This was mental torture for me; no hard-shell brace touching me, no straps holding me, all invisible but just as binding and even more controlling.

If I didn't know where the day's travels would bring us, I would place a cold rag in a thermal bag, so I could reapply it to her face. Keeping her hydrated while making sure she didn't aspirate was constantly on my mind. We welcomed any air-conditioning opportunities; but occasionally, when I had extra help, I would just opt to go to our local pool and take full advantage of removing the damn brace!

Now, snapping out of my daydream and back to reality, I rolled Jacklyn into the kitchen and sat down with my mother to have breakfast. There were bills and other mail staring at me from the opposite side of the table. I recalled how hurt I felt years ago, knowing many other families received the same letter regarding their child's brace and medical bill.

A few years ago

Periodically, as years passed, Jacklyn needed to be refitted four times due to growth and adjustments. The cost for each new brace was $600. We continued to use the same orthopedic provider. One evening, after reviewing the explanation of benefits on a new insurance bill, I noticed that the brace was now costing $1,800.

Occasionally, I had difficulty confronting doctors and some of Jacklyn's professionals with questions. But this time during our next visit, I asked, "Why was there a $1,200 jump in the price?"

He looked down while picking up one of his handiworks and said in a monotone voice, "The $1,200 increase was because I discovered Medicaid would pay more for it." I said nothing in return; I was speechless as I frowned at him, expecting another comment. With a serious, straight, frozen face, and avoiding eye contact, he left the room. As I rolled Jacklyn out of the office passing Cindy, Tommy, Julie, and Matt's braces, I was fuming, especially since I had heard Medicaid cuts services to save money. They cut crucial services and in turn hurt the people who need help the most! This was unethical and immoral! It goes against my grain, yet I was part of it!

Although this may have been legal to do, allowing the system to increase the payment seemed like stealing. He was getting more for the same service. What else would he do to get more? This proved to me that our government is not able to put a proper price on medical services and equipment. Medicaid loses money through fraud, but this was waste on the government's behalf. My life's daily battles were frustrating enough, and then, to be part of this was even more discouraging. In some way, I felt part of a crime and thought about those who'd been denied services because of limited Medicaid funds.

This upsetting situation haunted me, but I wasn't capable of fighting the entire system beyond voicing my opinion to the insurance company. I wished I had the energy but instead became complacent and just accepted the sad fact that this was government bureaucracy at its best! I thought about all those braces I saw in the orthopedic provider's office on my first visit and wondered if the parents of Cindy, Tommy, Julie, and Matt received this information and felt the same way.

AHRC Saturday Respite Program

Jacklyn liked to hear other children. Whenever she was in a doctor's office or a local park, or near any screaming or crying children, a tiny smirk would appear. She delighted in the commotion, and her eyes would widen with each child's howl. On one occasion, I needed to bring her to the pediatrician's office. There were many extremely loud children waiting, and Jacklyn turned toward the loudest group. With a smile, her hand to her mouth, she added to the conversation a "grrrrr," a pause, and then another "grrrrr." As she continued to act happy and alert, I didn't want to leave the office and go home. We were cheating her by not offering extra stimulation. Our home setting was limited. Repetitive music and physical therapy could become boring. I wanted her to have more.

I heard about a Saturday recreation program in a nearby town. I followed up and met with the respite program director at the Association for the Help of Retarded Children at Brookville. After giving a detailed medical background of Jacklyn, including her IEP (Individual Education Plan) and signing consent forms, I was still uneasy. "I will place Jacklyn with an excellent caretaker," was her reassuring comment. Upon leaving our meeting, I struggled to overlook my anxiety and my emotional baggage and not cancel the arrangement.

Jacklyn was developmentally equivalent to a one-month-old baby. If she wasn't constantly supervised, anything could happen. I didn't want to regret my decision. I was torn, not knowing how she would fit in. What kind of setting would she be placed into? Would it be with other non-verbal kids? Would she be the only one who couldn't see, walk, or talk? Would she be the only one who had a seizure disorder? Who would be able to read and understand her like I do?

I was pessimistic as Karl and I drove the lengthy winding road passing breathtaking mansions, a country club, and a large group of bicyclists. A long, low brick wall with a huge black gate marked the entrance to the AHRC complex. I didn't know how I was going to rip myself away from Jacklyn and leave her. Aware of my feelings, Karl turned to me and declared, "Let's give this a chance." We both agreed this was something positive for her, but my heart was still pounding.

We proceeded to park and noticed children, ranging from ambulatory to wheelchair bound, entering the building. "Hey Jacklyn, you are going to have a ton of new friends," I told her. As we slowly rolled along the path, I stopped to take in the beautiful view and wished Jacklyn could see the nature that surrounded her. The soft breeze took little strands of hair that escaped from her ponytail and whipped them across her face. Those few elusive hairs brushed against her eyelashes. After she gave me a cheerful grunt and happy grin, I removed the wisps of hair that tickled her face. "Okay, let's go. It's time to meet new playmates," I whispered.

The program director approached us with a large clipboard as we walked into the facility. "Good morning, Jacklyn. I've heard so much about you," she said as she touched Jacklyn's hand. She then turned to us and said that Jacklyn's presence ". . . spoke volumes." As I waited for her to check in the other children, I thought about that statement. *What did she mean Jacklyn's "presence spoke volumes"?*

The gym was being flooded with many yelling, excited special children along with a vast crew of volunteers and trained professionals. It was controlled mayhem that brought a grin to my face and Jacklyn's, too.

A stout young man with wire-rimmed glasses greeted me with a smile. "Hello, my name is Ricky, and I will be Jackie's primary caretaker."

"Hello," I replied. "Nice to meet you. Can I stay for a while?"

"Sure. Stay as long as you need," he replied while introducing himself to Jacklyn. "We can go over her braces, feeding, positioning, respiratory care, medication, likes and dislikes." I ended up staying for that session and the following few sessions as well.

This was a therapeutic, recreational respite program, and after a few weeks, I was the only mother still hovering!

As I retreated to a far-off corner, again quietly observing, I got the perception that Ricky was a caring, joyful, and genuinely kind individual who was extremely vigilant over his charges. He appeared to have a gift that not all caretakers possess.

Upon Jacklyn's next visit, I entered the gym upset. I knew what had to be done, but doing it wasn't easy. Ricky approached me and said, "You can leave her." I looked at him and nodded. He then commented, "Trust us."

As I kissed Jacklyn's cheeks, I said, "You be a good girl and have fun" and returned to my car.

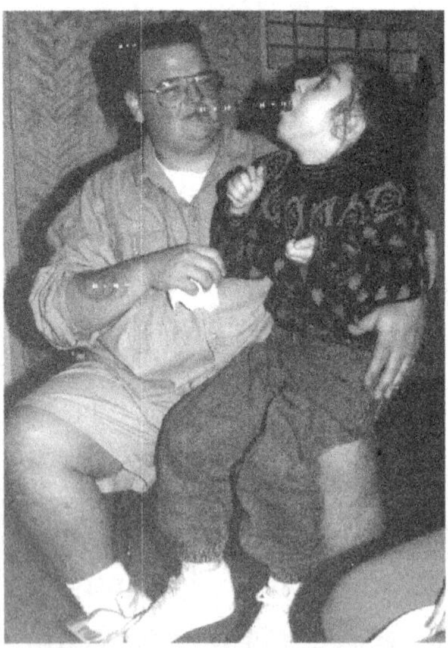

After a few months, Ricky confessed to me that Jacklyn had become a great communicator. I beamed at him just like a teacher would look at one of her students who understood the meaning of the lesson. He claimed she taught him how to listen and observe. I smiled, thinking back to when he asked me to "trust" and when I sensed he had that special gift—the ability to understand without hearing a single word.

A year passed, and it was getting close to Halloween. The staff had planned a Halloween costume party. Everyone was talking about what they intended to wear for that upcoming special respite. Upon reaching home, I fought my negative thoughts, those demons that entered my mind that could derail Jacklyn's opportunity to be part of the festivities. I asked myself, "What kind of costume can I find for my daughter who is in a wheelchair?" The challenge of her being different couldn't stop me. I wanted to come up with something extraordinary.

During the night as I tossed and turned, it came to me! I knew exactly what to do. The next day I went to a craft store and purchased a few yards of orange material and a bit of green and black to start my project. I worked on the costume every night until the outfit was perfect. During that time, I felt like any other mother who was preparing Halloween garb for her child. Cheerful and almost giddy to be doing a normal parental task, I wasn't a broken link in a chain.

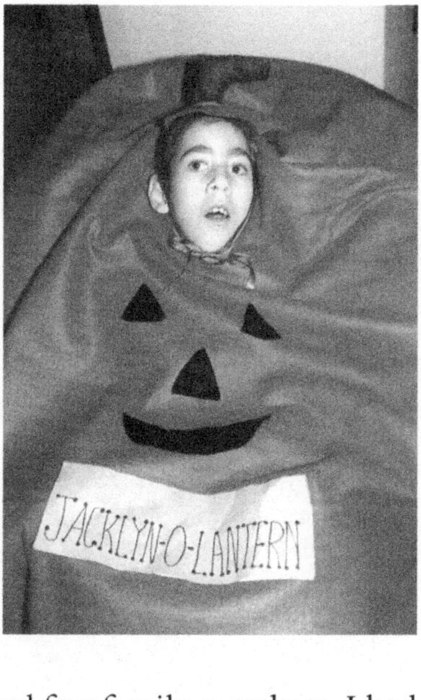

With my husband, mother, and few family members, I had the reveal the night before the AHRC party.

Jacklyn was going to be *JACKLYN-O-LANTERN*

I traveled that winding Brookville road to the AHRC center almost every Saturday for three years. Jacklyn's weekend routine, with her friends and trusted caretakers, was priceless.

I often wondered what she might be thinking. How much fun was this activity for her?

Upon leaving the play area that day, I kissed her softly on her cheek. She quickly turned to me with a half-smirk and made a little happy sound I'd heard before, which meant "I'm fine. See you later!"

Genetic Testing

I had expectations for myself on how to be a good parent. I learned during childhood by watching TV shows and mimicking my own family. *Ozzie & Harriet, Father Knows Best,* and *Lassie* depicted good family values. It's also human nature, motherly instincts!

I remembered the feeling when Jacklyn was placed into my arms after I'd given birth. My desire to give Karl, the love of my life, a child, to start a family together, had finally come true. Her weak cry and wrinkled soft skin amazed me. As I looked at Karl, he said softly, "She is perfect, has ten tiny toes, ten tiny fingers, and a lot of dark hair." Karl's beaming proud smile as a new father totally completed me as a wife.

Now she was almost five years old, and as her mother, I was still expected to fix all her problems. I must take care of her needs and wants, and protect her. I was supposed to do so, but, without a diagnosis, how was this possible? How could I follow the correct path—one that will give her the best quality of life and a chance to reach her full potential?

There were days I felt like a punch-drunk boxer—charging forward, getting hit, knocked down, and then getting up and repeating the process. My battle scars were not visible, they were hidden from the world. No one could see the cuts and bruises that were deep within my body. My trainer, aka Karl, was the only one who kept me going, because he believed in me. We were a team. Teamwork and motherly love had carried me to this point, but the fear of depression and falling into the abyss, unable to "claw and scrape" back up scared the hell out of me. I didn't want to be buried by the weight of a spiraling depression again. It could change everything in an instant.

Jacklyn had ups and downs but had always stabilized. She was still in diapers; she couldn't hold objects; she was fed pureed foods; she couldn't walk, talk, sit up, see, or stand. Having a brother or sister after your firstborn was normal for most families. But future children for us would be questionable. How could I bring another sick child into this world? It would be selfish! I could fail once again. But, watching the news and hearing reports of how new discoveries in medicine were helping various afflictions gave me hope. I dreamed and prayed for a miracle, a miracle of hearing the cry of a healthy newborn, an infant free of the horrible disease that robbed and confined.

All attempts to find an answer left me drained and frustrated. I was stuck, unable to move in any direction. It was a jail cell with bars that circled not only Jacklyn, but me as well. I was trapped in many ways—unable to produce a healthy child. My femininity was torn away and removed from my being. I was no longer looked upon to be a child-bearing female for the chance that I could produce another sick infant—damaged goods, useless when it comes to the family unit. I had failed as a mother by not finding a cure for my child. How could I love someone so much and let her suffer and not give her the life she should be living?

Sitting in this imaginary prison cell, the answer to the problem sits in an envelope right outside the long jail cell bars, but I can't reach it. Snatching that paper to pardon both of us was only an arm's length away. Finding a diagnosis for Jacklyn was critical. The desire ran deeper than just finding out for ourselves. It became a quest for knowledge that might help other relatives when they started a family.

Desperately wanting answers and with help from Jacklyn's new doctor, we pursued genetic testing. We planned to visit the Institute for Basic Research (IBR) in Staten Island. The appointment was set, and I felt optimistic but guarded. My shield and armor were always nearby.

It was the evening before the appointment. "Get me another towel," Karl shouted. "Lucille, please get another towel."

"Sure," I responded, quickly snapping out of being lost in thought about tomorrow's meeting. I went to the hall closet and got another bath sheet.

We were giving her a bath; she had become a two-person lift. Karl took her shoulders while I took her legs. Still wet, she is slippery, so we gently raised and removed her from the tub and placed her onto the long bath sheet that had been placed onto the bathroom floor. I slipped on the tile floor but regained my footing.

Karl said, "Are you okay? Be careful. Can you do this?"

"Yes, I can do this," I replied as I begin patting away the water and placing a smaller towel on her head and hair.

"Ready. Are you ready?" Karl asked. "Ready, one, two, three, and lift," he shouted as we lifted her in unison off the floor while holding tightly each corner of the long bath sheet. I was careful as I began walking backwards. I couldn't see her face as she swayed side to side, while Karl and I held the corners of the bath sheet. Her body was almost totally covered with the towel, into which she sank, as one would sink into a hammock. She swayed from side to side as we carefully walked until we reached her bedroom. Karl continued to do most of the lifting, and I wished I could do more. My back was stiff and sometimes gave me a shooting pain. Yet, he never complains. Never!

After I put Jacklyn's nightgown on her, Karl carried and placed her into bed. He kissed the top of her head while saying, "I love you," before giving me a kiss good night and saying, "I love you, too."

After he left, I whispered into Jacklyn's ear, "You have a very special daddy." I tucked her in. Then, I started to read a new book I'd bought that day—the type where you press a coordinated button when it appears during the story to hear a musical tune or sound. She listened to the different sounds and was content. Her eyes were getting heavy as she listened to the soothing music. I still wished that she could see the pictures—raising the book to place it close to her face right before she fell asleep.

The next day, we were up and on the road. After a two-and-a-half-hour ride, we reached the facility. Skin samples were taken from Jacklyn, and we were told it would take weeks to process. All I could think about on the return trip home was, *If there was just one scientist who could determine the cause, then we had a fighting chance.* Just one breakthrough, one new discovery, one doctor could change our world. Medicine could be created to help her and then give us the opportunity to have another child free from this disorder. It was possible!

A few months passed. Finally, the envelope arrived, and we sat at the kitchen table. I said, "Karl, you open it." His eyes were wide with anticipation as he removed the report. I stared at his face, looking for a sign of hope, studying every expression, and watching for any positive body language. As he turned each page, his lips read each word slowly to himself. He shuffled the papers back and forth and then removed one from the rest. Could this be the pardon I was hoping to receive? Karl's eyes lowered and then looked up at me saying, "They found inclusions in her cells, indicative of a storage disease. The workup was inconclusive."

Karl read further. It was leaning toward a class of *Neuronal Ceroid Lipofuscinoses*.[1,2] At this point, I slapped down the papers out of Karl's hands. Then I erupted. "What does *that* mean? What does *that* mean?" Karl reached over to me, and I continued, "They made a mistake. I'm calling our hospital tomorrow to get a second opinion."

I needed a second opinion, so we took her to the Genetics Clinic at the children's hospital. Again, the evaluation left us without a definite answer. They were not able to come up with a diagnosis or any further information. It was not possible for them to determine if the cause of her developmental arrest and

1 (See Wikipedia) Neuronal ceroid lipofuscinosis (NCL) is the general name for a family of at least eight genetically separate neurodegenerative disorders that result from excessive accumulation of lipopigments (lipofuscin) in the body's tissues. These lipopigments are made up of fats and proteins. Their name comes from the word stem *lipo-*, which is a variation on "lipid," or "fat," and from the term *pigment*, because the substances take on a greenish-yellow color when viewed under an ultraviolet-light microscope. These lipofuscin materials build up in neuronal cells and many organs, including the liver, spleen, myocardium, and kidneys.

2 (See National Center for Biotechnology Information) The neuronal ceroid-lipofuscinoses (NCLs) are a group of inherited, neurodegenerative, lysosomal storage disorders characterized by progressive intellectual and motor deterioration, seizures, and early death. Visual loss is a feature of most forms. Clinical phenotypes have been characterized traditionally according to the age of onset and order of appearance of clinical features into infantile, late-infantile, juvenile, adult, and Northern epilepsy (also known as progressive epilepsy with mental retardation [EPMR]). There is, however, genetic and allelic heterogeneity; a proposed new nomenclature and classification system has been developed to take into account both the responsible gene and the age at disease onset; for example, CLN1 disease, infantile onset, and CLN1 disease, juvenile onset, are both caused by pathogenic variants in *PPT1* but with differing age of onset.

seizures were genetic. Prenatal diagnosis for the recurrence of her disorder in a later pregnancy was not possible.[3]

Another failed attempt to find an answer. The jail cell door was permanently locked, and the key was thrown away, unless another plan was developed. The only alternative to eliminating the possibility of a 25 percent recurrence risk was through artificial insemination by a donor.

Time passed, and I realized that the longer we had to wait for a definite answer, the less of a chance there was that we could find a cause and potential cure for Jacklyn. The seizures had become less controlled. Some were seizures, and some were not. Believing that doctors had all the answers, could cure all sicknesses, give hope to the hopeless was truly a fabrication of my imagination. How could I have been so naïve?

I tossed and turned at night because the problem goes beyond us three. It was bigger than us. Eventually, Karl and I sat down one night after Jacklyn was asleep, and we both confessed the same sentiment. I said, "What about our relatives? How can they check and make sure the same or similar recurrence doesn't happen in their family? I wouldn't wish this nightmare on anyone."

Karl replied, "We are doing everything possible." I personally was exhausted, and, for now, we had hit a dead end.

---

3 The review stated that genes are the basic units of hereditary information—the code for proteins responsible for all body traits and characteristics. There are thousands of gene pairs in each cell—one pair (or two matching copies) codes for each trait. We understood that when an individual receives two copies of an abnormal gene, having inherited one copy from each "carrier" parent, a genetic disease results. Parents who carry the same abnormal gene have a 25% chance to have children affected with the disorder and a 75% chance to have unaffected children.

Thoughts about my biological clock and the fact it was running out had been more frequent. *Tick, tick, tick!* It was loud and clear. Accepting the fact that I was running out of time was a difficult pill to swallow. I'd failed at my one important job. Plus, I'd put Karl into this situation. I told Karl, "Everything I do for the first time is a failure." I reminded him how I was a failure when I attempted to breastfeed, too. He just shook his head and held me close, his plaid shirt absorbing my tears.

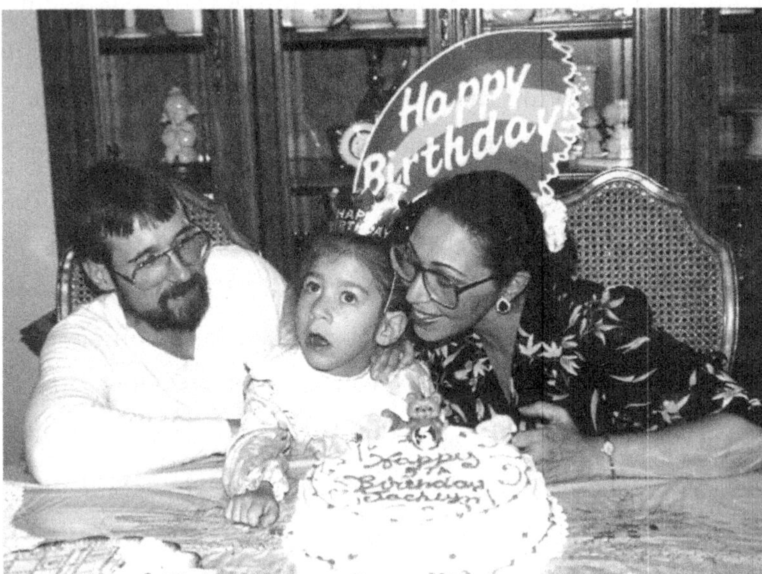

I realized that the next step for us would be either to adopt or try *in vitro* fertilization. From start to finish, either option would take us years, plus an emotional and physical toll. The decision had to be made as a family; it was not solely mine to make. Part of me had surrendered, and another part still had a small glimmer of hope. I continued secretly, without telling Karl, researching both options whenever time and energy allowed. Jacklyn's care and striving to stay mentally strong were my primary focuses. There was very little left of me to pursue the dream of Jacklyn having a sibling now.

Ferncliff Manor

Having to go through the motions of daily living is necessary. Shopping for food, doing laundry, paying bills, maintaining a home, and upkeep of a car continues. It's a fact that cars need to be replaced from time to time. I don't recall what the reason was, but we found ourselves in need of a new car. Karl cheerfully said, "Go pick one." I felt an adrenalin rush that put me on an emotional high. Karl and I spent evenings discussing the pros and cons of different cars. I escaped to a make-believe fantasy land where husbands and wives do fun chores—tasks of which they had control over the outcome. I thought, *Who wouldn't want a new car? This purchase might get me out of my rut.* Ultimately, Karl said that I should make the final choice.

I was energized with the anticipation that it would fix my mood and made a decision. After a brief instruction session on key mechanical features, I drove away in my shiny new black car. The smell of a new vehicle is something everyone remembers. The clean, crisp aroma tickled my nose as I slowly felt a smile creep up on my face. It felt strange to smile. I'd almost forgotten the physical mechanics of smiling. It had been a long time.

Making a left onto Euston Road South, I saw a young child making funny faces as she looked out from the rear window of her parent's car. I blinked, and suddenly the little face became Jacklyn, staring at me. Now, approximately one mile from home, the truth hit me and hit me hard—*bang!*—as if I'd driven into a brick wall and glass was flying in every direction! I broke out in a cold chill, my heart pounding so hard that I felt it over the vibrations generated from the car's stereo system.

This purchase was a material object, but reality was less than a mile away. It didn't and wouldn't change a damn thing. It was just a hunk of metal. It can't take away the pain, the anger. It's lifeless, just like I am at times, hollow and void of happiness. A machine, yes, just a machine. Just like me! Just like me! Half a mile away and with each passing block thereafter, closer and closer, the feelings of emptiness and meaninglessness overpowered me. Now, I could see my home and driveway quickly approaching. At this point, all I wanted to do was take this heap of metal back to the dealer but knew that was impossible.

As I pulled into the garage, where no one could see or hear me, I exploded, screaming and hitting the steering wheel with my fists—trying to beat and punch away this horrible situation. Then I pounded my head with my hands to stop my madness.

Still shaken, I walked into the house and tossed the keys on the kitchen table. Karl looked surprised, and I yelled, "This doesn't mean anything to me! Oh, my God! What have I done?"

Perhaps Karl thought this would help, but it had failed miserably. He knew we had bigger troubles ahead but still tried to console me by stating, "We needed a new car anyway, and it's safer for transporting Jacklyn."

How stupid was I to think I could move on and start living a normal life? Not today. No, not today. I nodded "Yes," as I held Jacklyn, telling her she had a new ride, describing the car to her, knowing she didn't understand and that she wouldn't be able to *see* it. She was stuck in her one-month world. Unable to see, talk, or walk. Stuck and not capable of moving forward. Locked in time. My beautiful child, so innocent, so vulnerable! Her lack of an expression said it all. I didn't notice her perk up as she often did when I talked in a happier tone. Did she sense the quaver in my voice, the sadness that I couldn't hide? I held her close until it was time for dinner, her head resting on my shoulder. Her arms hung limply down, unable to hold or hug me in return. As a family, we had other problems facing us. The car was a brief sidetrack from our next obstacle.

The lifting, changing diapers, transporting in the wheelchair up and down steps and carrying her at times has taken a tremendous toll on my back. Concern over her choking on saliva at night has compromised many nights of sleep. Karl's business trips were more frequent and took him away from home for days at a time. The pain and pressure had been building up.

We needed relief and applied through our school district for a residential facility. More sleepless nights, more discussions, more bouts of my insides hurting; but, reluctantly, we relayed our appeal. They approved and mailed us a list of potential options. I was tormented with the thought of her being away from home and my watchful eye. We were one being! I could sense most emotions and responded to her needs. A plan was devised in which she would be away for only a few days each week. By altering our work schedule, a viable solution was created. But the distance had to be reasonable for it to work.

We planned to visit some of the homes listed to evaluate their potential. What they had to offer was listed and reviewed with detail before we scheduled each appointment. We headed to one of the closest in New Jersey, about two-and-a-half hours away, barring any major traffic jams. I hated their lack of cleanliness, and the hospital-type feeling really turned me off. That was a short visit. I prayed that this was not going to be the norm for the remaining sites. Our second visit brought us upstate, approximately five hours from home. It was beautiful, with a complete sensory room filled with audio and other forms of stimulation. It was an immaculate campus, with a complete physical therapy program. It was fully staffed, with a good ratio for each child, but it was quite far away.

After visiting a few more facilities, a light had shone through, the rainstorm had passed, and a rainbow appeared. This light was bright over Ferncliff Manor in Yonkers, New

York. It had a children's school program, family involvement, therapy schedule, and activities. It was clean, close to home (within one hour) and was a family-operated facility with a caring staff. We chose Ferncliff as Jacklyn's new part-time home.

Jacklyn was now five years old. It was important for her to have loose-fitting clothing, otherwise changing her diaper would be more difficult. I was given a list of items to buy that included clothing for her Ferncliff home. Purchasing outfits for her wasn't the experience most mothers are blessed to have; no, it was quite the opposite. When I went to the children's clothing department, I always envied other mothers because they could buy fancy dresses, dress shoes, sandals, cloth coats, and hats. I couldn't. I was limited. I had to make sure elastic waistbands were on all of Jacklyn's pants. The pant legs had to be wide enough for the leg braces to fit comfortably. Socks had to be cotton and knee-high to cover her skin and shield them from the plastic leg braces. All her tops had to be oversized to fit over her scoliosis brace. All winter coats had to be of a non-absorbent fabric, so when she spits up, it could be easily cleaned. Shoes, a girl's favorite item, were not a major purchase; there were not many in her closet—just oversized sneakers and a few pairs of elastic slipper-socks.

Nevertheless, with a task that had to be accomplished, I purchased a few new functionally appropriate outfits that were as cute as possible. I dropped them all off at my mom's home. She helped by sewing Jacklyn's name labels onto everything—even socks—for her Ferncliff wardrobe. The little voice in my head said it was as if she were going off to camp. That calming voice was the one I listened to often. It's the same little voice that helps me put on my protective armor when I can't handle another problem. This voice belonged to one of God's guardian angels, who stood by all mothers who have children who are less than perfect. They must teach mothers like me that their child will live in his or her own special world. Helping each mother to be patient and recognize that if they are one of the lucky ones to hear a spoken word or witness a step, it was truly a miracle.

One doesn't realize the amount of time needed to place a name label on every piece of clothing. Thank God for my mother, aka "Grandma Mamie." She had the patience and skill to sew the clothing labels as well as to create many macaroni-and-meatball dishes. Over the past few years, I'd moved away from baby jars and would puree the pasta and meatballs, so Jacklyn could enjoy the Sunday meal with us. I learned how to puree almost any meal that Karl and I shared so that she would be totally part of our family dinners. Chopping pieces up into small chunks and then placing them into the mini-blender was a weekly routine. The blades would spin until I achieved the right texture before I tasted the final product. When I was satisfied with the texture and taste, I placed them into ice-cube trays and froze them. I knew a facility like Ferncliff would prepare a larger variety, and that certainly would be a plus for her. I had to focus on the positive and remind myself that it was only a few days during the week. She would hear other children, and have more caretakers and additional therapy. *It would be better for her. Just a few days. Just a few days.*

During check-in on one return trip, I provided an update on Jacklyn's weekend to the nursing staff. It was uneventful. I then wheeled her to Mary, who was Jacklyn's caretaker. She was a big woman with a big smile to match. She was soft spoken and had already lifted and cradled my child in her arms against her ample bosom. I looked at Jacklyn and sensed something was wrong. I couldn't figure out what was bothering her, but immediately I felt the guilt of leaving her and being so far from home. As I left the facility with my insides in knots, I drove down the hilltop to the main road. There, at a stop sign, with no other cars around, I shut my car off. Lowering my eyes and taking a deep breath, forced to understand things without the logic of words, my instinct told me not to continue. Like a trumpet blasting within me, signaling a warning, I turned around and headed back to my daughter.

Mary was still cradling Jacklyn and waiting to prepare her for a bath before bedtime. She was next in line. I approached Jacklyn and caressed her face. Her expression did not sit well with me. Mary helped me place Jacklyn back into her wheelchair, and I took her over to the nursing station.

My senses were right on, and, sure enough, she had a temperature. They put her on Tylenol. I returned home extremely late that night but felt thankful for being able to quickly diagnose my child in a way that no one else would be able to do.

As I tried to fall asleep after such a busy day, I thought about the other children who did not have family visitors. It haunted me that, earlier, an aide confessed to me that most of the children didn't receive visitors.

"No one?" I asked while the thought broke my heart.

She said, "No, not like Jacklyn." I figured one of the reasons was the fact their parents and/or family were too far away to make frequent trips. Other families had other children, who occupied their time; and compounding the problem, the distance made it impossible to visit often. Still, it was hard to comprehend because my weekly visits were a lifeline for my survival. That day I made a promise to myself that I would be more attentive to the other children with every visit. I never judged other parents, as I would not have wanted to be judged.

The nursing staff continued to monitor her for any temperature spikes and kept me updated as her condition improved. Since she was prone to aspiration and pneumonia, this required medication administered in a nebulizer. A mask was placed over her nose, allowing her to breathe the prescribed amount of medication in the form of a mist inhaled into her lungs. While she was being treated at home, I would watch this lifesaving vapor enter her body. The little mask around her nose would fog up with the healing vapor steam. It appeared to relax her, and, at times, she would fall asleep as I held her hand. I felt helpless to change what had now become another necessary medical intervention. I shook my head in disbelief when I reviewed her daily regime of medical requirements. An around-the-clock team is essential. I quietly said, "Things could be worse; things could be worse; things could be so much worse."

March 7, 1992, was approaching, and the excitement of the staff, children, and parents was mounting with each passing day. Ferncliff Manor was part of the Westchester-Putnam Special Olympics Junior Games hosted by The Masters School. We were told the morning began with the children being transported a short distance to the school gymnasium. After meeting the bus, I wheeled Jacklyn into the vast room that contained numerous signs. The commotion excited her, and she knew something different was about to take place. She turned to all the other children's happy shouts and added her own little hoot with half-smile. We were handed lunch and a schedule for the day by a young lady volunteer from The Masters School. She politely introduced herself while giving me a purple Special Olympic shirt for Jacklyn to wear.

The Special Olympic Games started after lunch, and I realized Jacklyn was going to have few opportunities to be involved because of her physical and mental limitations. Many of the participants had already been engaged in different events. Their thunderous laughter echoed in the gymnasium. I sensed her disappointment as she heard the commotion all round her as she sat strapped in her chair. I was not willing to give up and needed to think of how I could include her in the fun.

Thankfully, with the assistance of two young ladies, we located a board approximately three feet by four feet that was on wheels and six inches off the floor. It probably was used for transporting chairs or other items in the gymnasium. With

Karl's help, I carefully placed Jacklyn down on the board and rolled her up and down an area used for track racing. She reacted to the gentle vibrations by putting her hand over her mouth with excitement. Up and down, up and down, repeatedly we rushed her along the track as her eyes widened followed by a long "grrrrr." I knew by Jacklyn's expressions that this game was a hit.

This was a rewarding moment, and it filled me with satisfaction knowing I'd created a unique experience for her. I felt like I'd won my very own "Special Olympic Parent Who Would Not Give Up" award.

Later in the afternoon, more than a dozen staff members positioned Jacklyn, while in her wheelchair, in the center of the room under a huge, round nylon tarp. It looked like they were using a colossal multi-colored parachute. *Whoosh, whoosh.* Lifting the tarp up and down, they created a whirlwind, and the breeze pleased her to the point of a big smile. Her hair flew in every direction as she placed her hand over her opened mouth. *Whoosh, whoosh.*

Overall, this was a very good day, free of seizures, while experiencing a variety of stimulation. She was happy, and I couldn't ask for anything more. I tucked this nice memory away into the corner of my mind because I knew I probably would have to draw upon it in darker and scarier days.

We rolled Jacklyn along the scuffed gymnasium floor to start her return trip to Ferncliff. The yelling and cheering now was replaced with quiet talk and the sound of equipment being moved about. I couldn't stop thinking of the children left behind and those who'd attended without parental involvement. I'm sure some children had parents who could not participate in the Special Olympics because they lived far away.

Maybe someday this problem will not exist. The more medically involved and dependent a child has become should not restrict and limit where he or she can call home. Their care must always be close to family, not forced abandonment because there is a lack of suitable facilities near loved ones. We were lucky to travel only one hour from home. Many families have special children who are separated by hours and live in other states because they lack proper housing in their community.

I felt the heartache of all those distant mothers, fathers, siblings and grandparents. As I looked at each child's face who passed on their way back to Ferncliff, I knew each one had a family that was experiencing the same anguish from separation. I could see in their little faces the emptiness in their eyes by not having Mom, Dad, Grandma, or Grandpa with them today. My only regret was that I couldn't be, just for today, a mother to all of those in that situation, so they, too, could smile.

Hip

A routine visit turned out to be a revelation. I watched intently as the doctor meticulously examined Jacklyn's curvature and hips. She slowly explained while pointing, "See here, if her hip popped out, it would be painful, and the curve would become worse." I looked at Jacklyn's back but said nothing, only nodding to show I understood. I was weary, beaten down because I had no control. Now, at almost eight years old, her twisted body might need surgery.

Driving home from the office, I rehashed what had been explained. The bottom line repeatedly flashed, MAJOR DECISION—MAJOR SURGERY! Like a neon light on a billboard: MAJOR DECISION—MAJOR SURGERY!

I was glad she was home for the weekend but not looking forward to discussing and making another critical decision for her care. That night, when I placed her into the bathtub, I studied her curve and hips. My eyes followed the line from the back of her neck slowly down as it forked off, taking a path of its own. I didn't want to put her through this painful operation—plus, I could lose her. But could I live with myself if we didn't act?

As I leaned over the tub to wash her hair, I said, "Give me a sign. What do you want me to do?" I wanted any kind of signal to release me of the responsibility. I wished she could tell me how much pain she was experiencing in her hip. What was the level of her discomfort? Her blank gaze as she continued to listen to the running water was all I got. If she sensed the fear in my voice, she didn't give me anything—nothing to relieve my anxiety. Nothing! This was absurd, because what parent asks a child if they want surgery? Part of me wanted to make believe she understood, to be connected, but it was only the lie I told myself—a fabrication that my mind created at times to hide her vulnerability. I tried to read her, communicate in other ways, but this time, I got nothing. She was totally helpless, and we had to be 100 percent sure of every choice. We couldn't risk making any mistakes. I couldn't live with myself knowing I'd caused her unnecessary harm or even worse.

The following week we received a second opinion confirming the need for surgery. The date was set. I didn't have a good feeling, but what parent would, given the circumstances? I was constantly telling myself that this was a "normal" anxiety—if that's even possible.

My stomach was in knots as we admitted her for the operation. Her innocent stares, unaware of what was going to happen, were eating at me, burning my insides to the point I wanted to run, taking her away, far away from the pain that we were going to let happen. The fire in the pit of my stomach was relentless. I was going to let this happen, yes, let my pure, sweet, unsuspecting child have this surgery. As a small moan emerged from within me, I continued to watch as she looked upward toward the bright overhead ceiling lights. I wished I could explain to her how we felt, how much we love her, and that we were doing the best we can. How I would trade places with her if only I could. I moaned again. Only Karl's reassuring voice pacified my fears for a few seconds.

"It's going to be fine. Try to calm down. We trust both doctors, and we didn't want to put Jacklyn in an emergency-surgery situation." She was taken away before I could wipe away a bit of drool and hug her one more time.

We waited for the surgeon to appear. I paced the waiting room, picking up various magazines, only to turn to one article and read the first paragraph before getting disinterested and picking up another magazine. All I could recall was her pale little face, staring off with a surprised expression as they rolled her away. Karl looked troubled but comforted me by saying, "We chose good doctors, did our homework, and shouldn't worry."

I spotted our white-haired surgeon through the small window that separated the waiting room's double doorway. He was easy to spot even though the window was tiny. "Karl, get up. I see the doctor," I exclaimed, while springing toward the double doorway.

The surgeon soon emerged in his hospital scrubs and said, "It was a difficult procedure, but everything went well. She is in the recovery room." A huge weight quickly lifted from my shoulders. Quickly rushing to her room, my heart was pounding so loud that I could hear it above the music in the elevator. As we entered, she was still asleep and in a spica cast.[4]

This was a shocking picture. A full-body cast had been explained to me, yet seeing it was alarming. "My poor child—what have we done?" I said, looking at her encased in this long, hard white cast that started at her mid-section, immobilizing her hips and thighs. "How are we going to give her physical therapy to keep her lungs clear? How are we going to change her diaper? How are we going to feed her upright, so she does not aspirate?" I broke out in a wave of cold chills. Karl reminded me that we were informed and that trained nurses could handle our issues. The six weeks that Jacklyn had to be immobilized was going to be very challenging, far more than I expected.

After a few hours, Jacklyn woke up crying. I was frantic—almost hysterical—because she never cried. Not like this, never

---

4 A cast which includes the trunk of the body and one or more limbs is called a "spica" cast, just as a cast is called which includes the "trunk" of the arm and one or more fingers or the thumb.

A hip spica includes the trunk of the body and one or more legs. A hip spica, which covers only one leg to the ankle or foot may be referred to as a "single-hip spica," while one which covers both legs is called a "double-hip spica." A "one-and-a-half-hip spica" encases one leg to the ankle or foot and the other to just above the knee. Hip spicas were formerly common in reducing femoral fractures, but today are rarely used except for congenital hip dislocations, and then mostly while the child is still an infant.

In some cases, a hip spica may extend down one or more legs to only above the knee. Such casts, called "pantaloon" casts, are occasionally seen to immobilize an injured lumbar spine or pelvis, in which case the trunk portion of the cast usually extends to the armpits.

with this intensity. Guilt that we'd made the wrong decision consumed my every thought. I yelled for a nurse. "Jacklyn needs pain medication quickly, *right now*." I ran out to the nurse's station, begging them to hurry. Karl remained at her bedside trying to console her. I stayed overnight, getting some rest only when she dozed off. All the doctor's good intentions could not erase the helpless feelings I had as I witnessed her in such pain. I failed in my job as her protector.

Her hospital stay was planned for one week; then she would go to a rehab center for a few weeks before returning to Ferncliff. Complications set in; her temperature went up and down for days, and we feared pneumonia. We were now approaching week four. Each day Karl and I were a tag team. We took turns driving the forty-five miles to Westchester to feed, clean, and provide extra physical therapy. Trying to comfort her with music, kisses, and holding her hand was part of my routine. But not a single smile was ever noticed. The cutout for her diaper became impossible to keep clean. This is not what I had envisioned—not even close.

I knew she was in pain by her tossing and turning her head. She fussed to the point that her signals were very clear to me and the entire hospital staff. During the quiet moments I spent driving to the hospital, the haunting decision to approve the surgery would eat at me relentlessly. I woke up at night reliving seeing her in pain and yelling for medication to comfort her. She was in the hospital for one month until the doctor cut off the cast; then, she gradually stabilized. What had we done? Was it worth it? Only time would tell.

As I walked to my car after my visit, I noticed a huge white tent with countless rows of white chairs in front of a stage. A table with stacks of pamphlets and literature was nearby. I picked one up and walked down the center aisle to take a seat and read about the ground-breaking ceremony that was planned. It was a campaign to build a children's rehabilitation center at St. Agnes Hospital. I noticed on the back of the pamphlet that Mrs. Agnes Carvel was the honorary chairperson. And, Kathie Lee Gifford and Frank Gifford were part of the celebrity council. That made my day. It restored my faith to know there are good people out there who want to help all these children. Lord knows I didn't have the time or energy. I loved Carvel ice cream and admired Kathie and Frank Gifford.

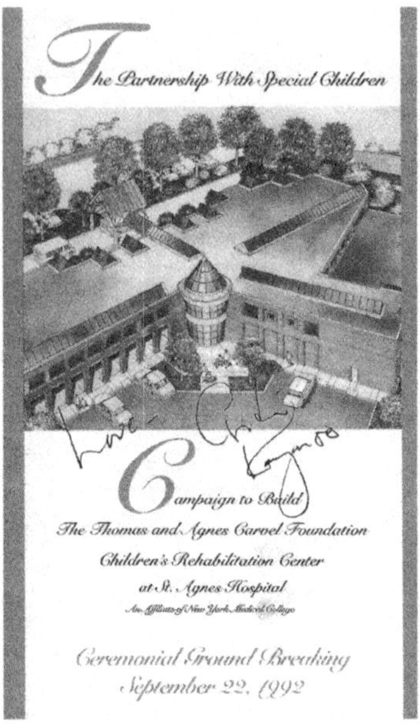
The Partnership With Special Children
Campaign to Build
The Thomas and Agnes Carvel Foundation
Children's Rehabilitation Center
at St. Agnes Hospital
Ceremonial Ground Breaking
September 22, 1992

Then, twenty feet in front of me, I noticed a man standing alone, facing the stage. He had a round face and was wearing a dark suit. Walking closer, I recognized his squared haircut with bangs and a walrus-type mustache. He was a childhood legend. I'd grown up with this soft-spoken famous TV celebrity.

I said, "Captain Kangaroo?"

"Yes," he replied as he turned to greet me.

Cheerfully I asked, "Where is Mr. Green Jeans?" He laughed and said he wasn't here with him today. We talked as I informed him of Jacklyn's hospital stay. As I explained her plight, he looked at me; his sad eyes told me more than any comforting words could. I confessed to him that I hoped Jacklyn would be released before her upcoming eighth birthday on the 25th. I wished him luck on the fundraising event. As I walked away, my emotions were running in every direction: high for having met him and then low for the fact that Jacklyn would never get the chance to appreciate this type of childhood joy.

The Phone Call

I was tossing and turning; then Karl gently shook me to wake up. I started sobbing and confessed that I'd had the same reoccurring dream. It was a replay of the scene when I was hopeful and optimistic, and the doctor callously told me, "Her brain waves are abnormal. Her life expectancy would be short, probably only a few years." Then, abruptly, he left the hospital room because he had prior dinner plans with his wife, leaving me to fall apart, ripping the little hope I had out of me. I can still hear the metal railing of Jacklyn's hospital bed clanging, echoing as I held onto them, trembling. I could still feel the cold steel in my hands.

Karl wrapped his arm around my shoulder to pull me close, saying, "We're doing everything possible." I heard him, but knowing she has a form of neurological degenerative disease and living each day for the doctor's predication to come true, and never knowing when it could all end was not really "living." I wanted to be with her constantly—every minute of the day and night. I wanted her to feel my presence, feel me close, know I'm there to protect her.

I tried to go back to sleep, but the guilt I felt over our separation stopped me. *I'm an awful mother to give up my helpless child, to be separated from her. It's forced abandonment!* My insides were ripping, and I wanted to distract myself. I went into the living room and paced, walking around the oval coffee table—around and around. I stopped briefly at the side table that held all my favorite family photos. Now, I continued to pace, but I held framed pictures of my dad and Jacklyn close to my heart. This pacing was not ridding me of my anxiety, doing little to offset the guilt. I couldn't stop thinking of what Jacklyn was doing this very second. Is she sleeping, or is she also awake? Could she be listening for me to approach to be at her side? Next, I sat on the couch and started to rock. All of this did little to tire me. I contemplated taking a sleeping pill but was fearful of where that road might lead. Before I returned to bed, I went to the pantry and checked to make sure I had an ample supply of Merlot and Chardonnay.

Morning came, and as I sat at the kitchen table, I was tired, barely keeping my eyes open. We were both up and getting ready for the day. The house was quiet except for the clanking of spoons and plates. I was staring at Karl as we were having breakfast. The previous night was one of my many nightmares. I looked at him and thought how blessed Jacklyn is for having him as her dad and how fortunate I am for having him as my husband, my supportive partner. I'd heard about many fathers leaving because they were unable to cope. Jacklyn has a father who is loving, caring, and dedicated. He had never been distant, removed from the crisis and leaving the burden totally on me. I didn't know what I would do without him. He has handled the mountainous medical bills, but, most importantly, he has been involved with every aspect of her needs. He doesn't approach it emotionally like I do, but logically. I guess all his computer training has paid off.

Yet, as logical as he tends to be, I captured moments of them together that showed his tender side. Many a night as I peered out of our bedroom to across the hall, I would catch him at her bedside, reading her a story book. Then he'd kiss the top of her head, saying, "Daddy loves you" before pulling up the covers and tucking her in.

As we finished our breakfast, I wondered if he was annoyed about last night. I told him I was sorry for waking him up. "Are you angry at me?"

There was a long pause while he placed the breakfast dishes into the sink. He told me "No" and that I should take a nap when I return home because he would barbeque dinner for us tonight. I smiled, giving him a hug. I was looking forward to this simple dinner, realizing I must try harder to be a better wife. I couldn't fail at this, too. I secretly wished I could be more like him.

Lately, there hadn't been a day that had gone by without my mind going through a mental rant: Why couldn't there be more facilities closer to home, where I could visit daily? As her mother, not her caretaker, I yearned for that maternal fix—to hold her in my arms. Nothing can replace the feeling and reassurance of seeing with my own eyes that she is fine.

Why do families have to be separated, hours away from their children? Again, I sensed this is forced abandonment! After my rant, I reminded myself that I knew it was getting dangerous to keep her at home. She needed to be in a 24-hour skilled nursing care facility. Whatever issue was being thrown at me, I had to realize that the problem or distance could be worse. Yes, so much worse.

She was back at Ferncliff at that time, but she could have been placed out of state. I had been informed that not every facility can handle all medical needs. Placement in another state—unthinkable! A four-hour one-way trip would make it impossible for reasonably frequent visits. If that happened, would I have to move, rent an apartment, drain our finances? Would we have to leave our jobs? What would happen to our medical coverage? Any loss in medical coverage would jeopardize Jacklyn's care.

I was afraid. That scenario would be a total defeat for us as a family. For now, I had to stop thinking. I felt like a puppy chasing its tail. It wasn't going to get me anywhere. I'd always tried to plan. Now I was responsible for my child, a special child. I couldn't think about this situation anymore. Worrying was only paralyzing me to the point that I was unable to function. Mental blockage of my daily concerns had become another job. That day was just another day that I must pick myself up, for her and for my marriage's sake.

One morning the telephone started ringing. One, two, three. It was going on the fourth ring, and I ran and picked it up just before it began recording on voicemail. "Hello,

hello," I said while I tried to catch my breath. I recognized the voice—it was Jacklyn's nurse from Ferncliff.

"Your daughter was rushed to the hospital by ambulance. She had difficulty breathing."

In a flash, I got the address and didn't ask any other questions. My mind raced. Could this be it? I grabbed my coat and pulled at Karl as he was entering the room. "We have to go *now*!"

As I was explaining to him, we both rushed to the car, and he started driving. Karl looked frantic. I needed to hear his logical predictions or calming comments, but I got nothing. He was driving with a wild look in his eyes, glued to the road straight ahead. He was unsettled and gripping the steering wheel so tightly that I thought it was going to break in his hand. I knew he was thinking the same terrible thoughts that I was visualizing. My heart was pounding. I could feel it beating in my chest as if it were going to burst. I placed my hand over my heart. I was starting to hyperventilate.

There was a traffic accident ahead of us, but we luckily cleared the area with ease. It didn't appear that anyone was hurt, but, honestly, I didn't care. I had little to no concern. I'd lost empathy. I thought back to all the times we'd attended supportive counseling sessions and listened to other parents' stories, only for us to be the worst case when it was our turn to share. I was empty inside. What had I become? My mind, my being, my every conscious moment could focus only on the brutal fact that Jacklyn, my child, was *not* close to home. She was separated from me, from us, who recognize what she needs without a word spoken. I ached, wondering what was going through her mind. Was she scared, thinking that we'd abandoned her? This was torture for all of us. This distance was cruel, callous punishment for being different.

I was rocking back and forth while babbling. Karl was not paying attention to my mumbling, my praying, my cursing, my love/hate relationship with God. "Why? Why? Just take me instead!" My shoulders were tense and hurt to the point I couldn't sit up straight. I felt pins and needles across the top of my back. I turned on the radio to try to break out, to escape, to rest my body. I was going to need all my wits when we arrived at the hospital. *What decisions would I be asked to make? I'll rely on Karl, but wish I were stronger.*

My mind went blank, shielding what I cannot or do not want to accept. I hate it, and yet I feel comforted when my mind shuts down and wraps itself in its own protective armor that feels like a warm blanket, hiding from the evil outside, numb to any negativity. I knew what I needed and should do as I stared out the window helpless. "It's all in God's hands." I hate my position, hate that my dreams are shattered, hate that my innocent child's life could end at any moment. Hate that she is suffering and that we, as her parents, are powerless. This is a never-ending, stomach-turning, tense, emotional roller-coaster ride. Every second that passed was filled with fear as to what we would discover when we arrived. I felt nauseous and found a small paper bag in the car.

Karl said, "Try to keep it together. We need to get there and don't have time to make any stops. If you have to throw up, do it outside the car window."

Now I could tell he was nervous, too, and needed to focus on driving—not on me. *Pull it together, pull it together!* I tried to calm myself by praying and repeating to myself, *This situation is out of my control.* I replied to Karl, "I'll try, but what happens if we get there and she is already gone?"

I dreamt of calm waters, wanting to feel my body floating downstream, not this stormy turmoil, tumbling over and swirling around, possibly drowning; having to fight the choppy waters with my arms violently thrashing and coming up for air only to be pushed down with each passing wave. I needed the soothing, peaceful calm of everyday life without constant fear. How I envied those families who drift along, oblivious to the beauty of their ordinary, simple life—to see their child walk, to hear them talk. What I would give to be ordinary!

Oh, would we be too late? Too late to say goodbye? Too late to hold her one last time? Too late to have her know that Mommy and Daddy loved her unconditionally?

The entire commute to the hospital, my stomach was in knots. I silently prayed with each passing mile. I thought, *God, she is in your hands.* Finally, we arrived, and Karl parked at the entrance. I bolted past the attendant, directly into the emergency room. "Where is my daughter?" I shouted.

We were directed by the staff to a bed with a full-length burgundy hospital curtain totally drawn around, encircling and blocking our view. Taking Karl's arm, I pointed to the floor. There were five pairs of shoes peeking out below the curtain. Five doctors and nurses huddled around her bedside. Almost the entire emergency room staff was at her side. *Oh,*

God—this can't be good, I thought. Shaking his head, Karl looked distraught and said, "Go ahead—open the curtain."

I called out, "Jacklyn, Jacklyn," while slowly sliding the drape. I held my breath as I reached out for Karl's hand for support. Then we both tugged at the material, peeking around the staff at her bedside. *Could this be it?*

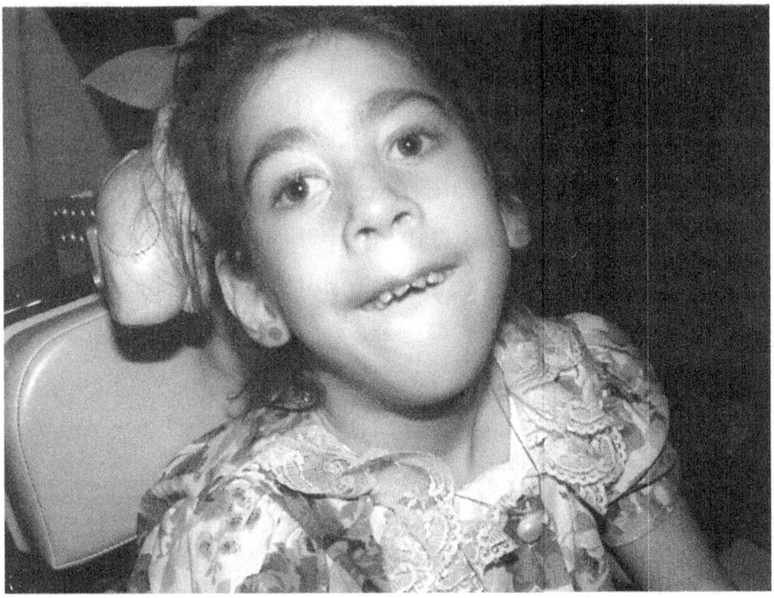

Jacklyn must have heard our voices. As we opened the drape, to our surprise, she greeted us with a smile. She turned to our voices and had a pleasant expression that I've seen so infrequently—placing her top teeth over her bottom lip with the corner of her mouth turned up into a smile. Then, she gave out a little happy grunt, which to me meant, "What took you so long to get here?"

Exhaling in relief, I laughed and cried at the same time. I felt like someone had shot me up with morphine, my body relaxing to almost numb. I scanned to see what had been done to her. I was surprised to see her red sweatsuit, cut off and lying near her feet, probably removed by the technicians in the ambulance. I could see the jagged scissor marks that ran directly up the center of her sweatshirt. I tried to dismiss the images of what had happened in the frightening ambulance trip and how Jacklyn couldn't communicate with them. After inspecting her chest and arms, I was content to see no major surgical intervention. I started kissing her face while wrapping my arms around her body, hugging her.

After speaking to the doctors, Karl put his hand on her head, stroking her hair and telling her, "Mommy and Daddy are here now."

I confessed, "Oh, Jacklyn—you aged me ten years." I was relieved she'd bounced back and was fine—this time!

Hospital Release; Then the Harley

The hospital released her after an evaluation and no signs of breathing difficulty. Pneumonia was our biggest worry. We signed the normal paperwork and took her home for the rest of the weekend. The remainder of the day was spent relatively free of any major medical issues.

The next day was clear and warm, and the birds fluttered about the huge tree in front of our home. I opened many of the windows to let in the fresh air, letting her hear the natural sounds of our world, the noises we pay little attention to daily. There were bugs bouncing off the screens on the front windows—maybe to avoid being eaten by the families of birds occupying the tree on our front lawn. Under our window, we could hear the squeaking wheels from a white-and-pink toy car as a child pedaled alongside her parent for a morning walk. I could smell the clippings of new grass, too.

I took a deep breath, feeling tranquil, and thankful for another day—for us, for her. I wanted the rest of our time together as a family to be happy, making what was left of our weekend more ordinary. I had a goal to try to make a normal day out of a *not* very normal life.

Later that day, Karl took advantage of the nice weather. "I'm going outside to wax the motorcycle and check the battery," he declared. Within seconds after hearing the garage

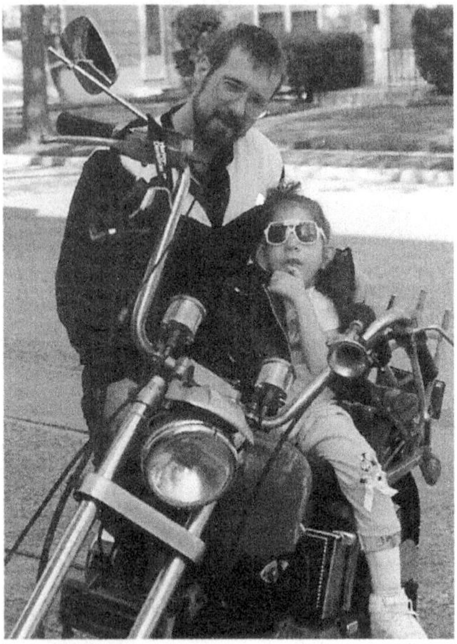

door open, there was that distinctive Harley engine roar. Jacklyn perked up upon hearing the sound and vibration outside our door. Seeing that, I dressed Jacklyn up in a little black jacket and placed toy sunglasses on her face.

"Karl, come get your little biker girl," I yelled from the upstairs window. As he entered the house, his smile said it all. He carefully carried Jacklyn and placed her on the massive seat of the Harley. One thing for sure, she loved the vibrating motorcycle when Karl cranked it up. I watched as he placed Jacklyn's hand on the throttle and turned it on. Her opened mouth, and her raised eyebrows showed her excitement. Then, raising her free hand to her mouth, she made a happy sound and turned in Karl's direction.

I had to mentally save this, a snapshot to place in the corner of my mind. Watching them involved in such a simple task, father and daughter sharing a simple moment, was beautiful.

As I was standing in the driveway, I could see behind Karl and Jacklyn, directly across the street. It was a father and his children walking back from the boulevard, probably returning home from the local playground. Yes, a mundane, ordinary chore. One of his children was driving a little white-and-red toy car, and the other older child was riding a pink bicycle with training wheels. I could hear the faint sound of the bicycle bell ringing, followed by a giggle from this toddler. I stared at him with envy—*this father doesn't realize how beautiful this everyday task is and how it should be cherished as a gift. Because it's not something that's guaranteed.*

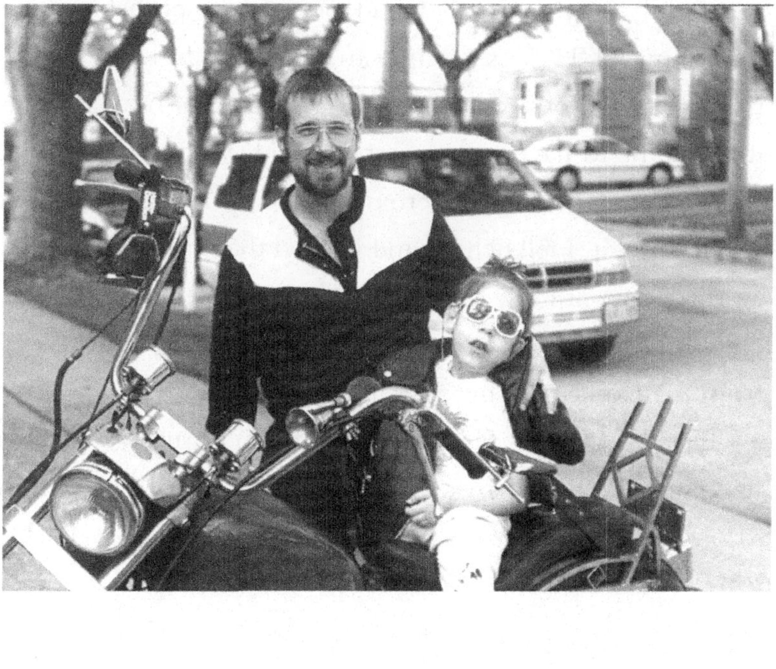

We had one more full day before returning Jacklyn to Ferncliff and decided to take her on a day trip to the Bronx Zoo. The smells and sounds would be great stimulation for her, and I couldn't resist experiencing this adventure, like other families.

We arrived, entered the park, and headed over to the bird sanctuary. It was calming and soothing strolling along the exhibit. It was a bit damp but full of life. The climate-controlled temperature and the chirping was relaxing for all three of us. As the birds fluttered around, Jacklyn's attention beamed upward. She raised her right hand and placed it at her mouth, then "grrrred" with amusement. I whispered to her, "You can fly like your bird friends the next time I take you on the park swing."

As we started passing through other exhibits, I noticed this one family—a mom, a dad, and a small boy, probably about four years old. He was running around, very excited to see all the animals. I looked at them and dreamed of how glorious it would be to have such an active child. We were different, and yet, as a family, we were the same. As I lingered longer at one exhibit, I fell behind and viewed them from a distance. At this moment I saw two families, both with happy children enjoying the zoo and Mother Nature, each child delighted from the experience but in their own unique ways.

Then it happened. Karl and I were taken by surprise. Jacklyn had a few small seizures. One right after the other. Within seconds of the onset of the first, another appeared. I was quickly yanked back to reality. We decided to take a seat under a tree until she recovered from the episode. My peripheral vision noticed that this young boy passed us again, but this time, he stopped and glanced over at Jacklyn in her wheelchair.

It was soon time for us to leave and return Jacklyn to Ferncliff. We started our long walk down the path to the parking lot. Suddenly, as we approached the lot, I heard the footsteps of a child running coming from behind us. I turned to look. It was the same family with the young boy. The parents were about twenty feet behind as the boy raced by us. After he began getting too far ahead, his dad yelled to him to stop, which he did. I could see he was observing Jacklyn with great concern.

Karl gave him a smile, and then the boy looked up at Karl and asked in a very curious tone, "Is she alive?" Stunned, my mouth dropped, but Karl, the cool-headed, devoted father that he is, just explained she was alive but was very tired. This was an innocent question from a young, inquisitive boy. The mortified parents overheard and took him aside. I watched his mother kneel, brush the hair away from his face, and speak to him. I could tell she was gently explaining while glancing over to us, mouthing, "I'm sorry." She chose to make this an educational moment. Who knew a trip to the Bronx Zoo could teach a child about Mother Nature and human nature, too?

As we walked to our car, I placed my hand on Jacklyn. She was still resting. I felt wounded, but this was different. My mind floated back to many years ago, when I took her for holiday photos at a local department store. I recalled another mother shielding her children's faces so that they couldn't see Jacklyn. If only more mothers explained the differences in others, then there could be more acceptance of those who are different. Maybe times have changed. I hope they have for the children's sake.

One Step Back

Tests, tests, and more tests. Earlier Karl went with the technician for Jacklyn's last test of the day. I was tired, and my stomach was rumbling. Eight years of going in and out of hospitals. Had I become accustomed to the routine? Eight years—yes, eight years—and they thought she would live only a few. We had become warriors; we fight, rest, regroup, and then fight again.

I was waiting, sitting in a small side chair in her hospital room, staring at the blank TV screen. I can't think about what the tests will show. Whatever it might be, she would bounce back. She always did. Each time I thought she would die, she bounced back. Why, for so many years, were we being dragged through this? There must be a reason. A dark cloud was hanging over us, and I wanted it to move on. But, when? When? It would be terrible for me to wish another family a challenging time. I'm a rotten person for letting that thought enter my mind, but this cloud needed to find another place. I wanted to be happy, free of constant worry. Free of daily contemplating a gloomy future. I didn't think it was too much to ask.

It was late in the afternoon, and the hospital floor that we were on showed few signs of activity. A low beeping sound was coming from the room across the hall. Nurses were quietly talking as they walked past our doorway. I could smell the food coming from the dinner cart that was delivered nearby. There was an occasional faint cry from a child in a distant room. The hall clock must have been broken, because time was standing still. I was nervous, and I needed to know the outcome, the verdict.

Soon they returned, and I could tell by Karl's appearance that the news wasn't good. His haggard face, ruffled hair, and weary, glazed-looking eyes told me more than words could say. Those once-shiny, very bright, delightful blue eyes now told me a different story. The hospital staff left the room, and Karl and I talked about this new turn of events. "I saw it with my own eyes. The test showed liquid entering her lungs, and that is one of the reasons she keeps getting pneumonia," Karl declared.

Still sitting, I shook my head. "*No!* What next?"

Half an hour passed, and our doctor arrived and explained. "I'm sorry to say, but Jackie is at an enormous risk. Please consider my proposal. A gastric feeding tube that goes directly into her stomach is one of two procedures to focus on better nourishment, calorie intake, and trying to keep liquids from entering her lungs." He paused and then urged, "Get back to me *soon,* because the surgery could be performed tomorrow."

I guess I will never understand how doctors can calmly deliver this type of medical news to profoundly stressed parents. Don't they look at the overall picture? I didn't want this operation to happen. Will this hurt her each time she needs to be fed? The human experience to eat and enjoy the flavor of different foods will end. She is a human being, not a machine. She has senses. She doesn't have much going for her, and the different textures and tastes were some of the good things in her life. How much more can be taken away from her and myself?

I didn't want to lose the close contact I had when feeding her pureed meals and thickened liquids. Thinking back, I couldn't breastfeed—all my attempts failed. I eventually gave up the effort. Now, with this, I'll have less contact, another failure. Mealtime was special to me. That was my exclusive time to look into her eyes to see if I could notice any interaction, any glimmer of connection, any happiness or contentment. Gone! Yes, gone, removed, taken away! No more patting her back or giving my circular rubs to get little comforting burps followed by her cute smile. Oh, it would be the slightest of smiles. Turning the sides of her mouth up ever so faintly. Then her eyes would close, content, having enjoyed assorted flavors and with a full belly.

Karl said while holding my hand, "Listen, we have to say 'yes' to this *now*. She is underweight and is prone to pneumonia." We talked, and I suggested getting another opinion. He continued, "We both have to agree on her care. It has to be a joint decision." He looked confident and then said, "Do you really want to put her through another test—even after I witnessed the fluid entering her lungs?"

I shuddered to think what could happen if I didn't give my permission. How could I live with myself if my poor judgment caused me to lose her now? There wasn't any room for mistakes. My tortured mind needs rest, an escape from life-and-death decisions that are always present. I must trust in Karl and the doctor's better judgment and know that this next step in Jacklyn's care is the right path—but it's so difficult to accept. I'm always holding out for something better, for a miracle.

As I listened to Karl, I knew he was right. He was always right and has been my rock all these years. When they say, "for better or worse," this was our "worse," and he hasn't run away from the commitment. I'm aware of many families with special children breaking up. I'm lucky to have him at my side, my partner.

Finally, I said, "Yes, Karl. You're right. Tell them to arrange the surgery as soon as possible." Kissing Jacklyn, I said, "I'm sorry—this has to be done." As we prepared to leave the hospital, I was upset. I didn't like the new path we were being forced into traveling.

I tried to get some rest and focused on how thankful I should be for Karl's patience and strength. There had been times when he'd had to re-explain to me repeatedly a doctor's instructions because I had put up a mental block and couldn't remember. Jacklyn and I wouldn't have made it this far on our own.

Before surgery, Karl sat me down and assured me one more time: "This is the right thing to do. Don't worry. I'll worry for the both of us." The procedure was performed the next morning without any other complications. My little girl, just eight years old, now had a permanent feeding tube in her stomach. After the surgery, I found it difficult to look at her belly—turning away whenever I accidentally caught a glimpse. I'd witnessed so much during our frequent hospital trips that I should have been stronger.

I thought that healthy children grew up and started feeding themselves. The key word here is feeding *themselves*, not a machine feeding them, not mechanical intervention. As I opened the 24-can case of liquid that would now be her sole source of food, I hurt—another dream crushed. This was just another milestone trampled into the ground. I could faintly hear from the living room the TV commercial advertising children eating their McDonald's Happy Meals. Damn, what awful timing!

That day was the first time I poured the can of liquid into the clear feeding bag. It was a beige liquid, missing any noticeable smell to speak of or any thickness in texture—bland and absent of how food tantalizes a person's appetite. Staring at the pole, bag, feeding pump, and Jacklyn, I hesitated. It was going to be a mechanical act, void of the warmth and emotions I had treasured. Hooking up the bag of liquid gave me a chill, just like the cold action I was about to perform. *I can't do this. Not this way.* She deserved more—yes, so much more. Grabbing one of our favorite musical books, I sat next to her, holding her hand and reading as the machine pumped away.

The next day I found Disney and *Sesame Street* stories on tape. I knew she loved to listen to the funny voices. I bought Disney's *Mary Poppins* and *Winnie the Pooh, Sesame Street*'s *Vegetable Soup* and the *Sesame Street Pet Show*. Her eyebrows would raise, and her eyes would widen upon hearing the Chipmunks singing songs. I relished every one of these moments that brought her happiness. Other days, when we had an opportunity to have dinner at the same time, we rolled Jacklyn and her equipment into our small kitchen. In time, Jacklyn started to gain weight and tolerated the change well.

A few weeks passed, and one day we were invited to a child's birthday party. I was watching other children feed themselves. Witnessing this stung and nipped at me. I found myself staring at them for a long time, transfixed, studying the mechanics of the diverse ways each child would hold a spoon. Others would just use their hands. One little girl focused on a single Cheerio and slowly swiped it up to her mouth. Two other toddlers placed more food onto their faces than into their mouths. What I would give to see Jacklyn attempt those actions! I continue to watch, hoping—even visualizing—my dream coming true. The visualization would overlay each child with Jacklyn's face, only for the image to disappear in a puff of smoke. But, even from this, I received a moment of contentment, satisfying a longing even though it could not be.

Aware of the amount of time that had elapsed, I got flushed with embarrassment. Had anyone noticed me staring? My face felt red hot, and I forced myself to look away. I scanned to see if anyone had caught me spying. My eyes darted back and forth until I was satisfied that no one realized. My secret was still intact. I controlled my desire to yell how fortunate they were. These parents had no idea the gift they were witnessing. I kept my thoughts to myself, deep inside, because I wasn't looking for pity. I had to ground myself. I didn't see Karl acting different around the other children—a perfect example of a good person, father, and husband. *Why can't I be more like him? Why? Why do I torture myself? Look away—just look away.*

I sat next to Jacklyn, holding her hand and hoping she enjoyed hearing the other children yelling. We were both quiet and in our own world, separate from the festivities that surrounded us. We were different! Luckily, she didn't feel the difference like I did.

Jacklyn has benefited by many lifesaving techniques that have come with all the medical advances. I repeated my mantra, quietly, to myself, *Things could be worse. Things could be so much worse.* I focused on the fact that she was filling out and gaining weight. She was no longer underweight. This was all good news. But I couldn't dismiss or totally erase the thought that it was getting more difficult to lift her. I couldn't avoid thinking about her future and ours. I was scared. She was growing, and we were getting older.

The feeding pump was easy to use, and the formula was delivered directly to our home on a regular basis. The medical supply company shipment packing invoice listed the 24-can supply as $120. Everything was paid in full by the insurance company.

During a local shopping trip, I happened to notice the *same* item at our local pharmacy. I checked and rechecked the labels and codes on the cans. The exact same formula—24-can supply. The case that our insurance company paid a hefty $120 for, according to our last bill, was listed as only $40, and it was the regular store price. This was crazy!

I called the insurance company and informed them of the dramatic difference in price. I offered, "I'll buy the case at the pharmacy, and you can then reimburse me."

They said, "*No!*" The representative explained, "It would be considered over-the-counter and not prescription." If we did this, we would be responsible for paying the $40 per case. Once again, bureaucracy at its best! This was obviously wrong and wasteful. Why does being different have so much extra baggage?

Scoliosis Brace

Another doctor's appointment! We were in the car, driving Jacklyn to her routine physiatrist visit. Most of our social activities as a family had become these follow-up trips or meeting new doctors for recent problems. Each doctor's appointment brought me to another level of concern, anticipating change. This time I was sweating—the clammy sweat that soaks you, and then you get chills. The exam could be good—it also could be bad, very bad. I hoped for the status quo—no change, no problem!

I recalled our first appointment. The doctor appeared knowledgeable and meticulous, and she was soft-spoken as she described how Jacklyn needed a scoliosis brace. She continued by explaining that, otherwise, her ribs would collapse her lungs as she grew. I never forgot that meeting or her advice. I didn't want it then; I didn't feel she needed it. Jacklyn was so small that I didn't even notice a problem with her spine.

Eventually, we went through eight new braces. Eight—that's eight changes—and she wasn't even ten years old. I have watched her pale little body be fitted again and again to help her grow straight. I should be accustomed to the ritual. I tell myself just that, but I'm *not*. It's funny how you can lie to yourself and almost believe it!

As I dressed Jacklyn that morning before her appointment, I traced my finger along until it curved off. I wished that my finger could miraculously straighten the bend—recalling how this doctor would take my hand to follow the length of her spine. She would show me how it still had taken a bit of its own path and direction. Knowing she was missing muscle tone, I gently massaged her, praying for better results, even if she had to get another new casting. I got a sick feeling in my stomach when I thought what her back would have looked like if she hadn't had a body brace for all these years. Oh, how that would have been a terrible, horrific mistake. I had to think like a fighter, a boxer in a ring. This was our fight, waiting for the bell to ring, dodging jabs, at times getting clobbered, dancing around the ring, giving us another round to survive.

We were called into an exam room after a short wait. When the doctor entered, we gave her a brief medical update since our last appointment. She examined Jacklyn and then looked at us and sighed. Waiting for what seemed an eternity for her to speak, I was getting nervous; she was being even *more* meticulous than usual. She was aware that Jacklyn had been experiencing more episodes of pneumonia and having trouble breathing. I tried to study her face but couldn't reach any conclusion. She exhaled. Then I stared at Karl, and he looked troubled, but he put his hand out to gesture for me to be patient. *How can he be so calm? Why is she examining in such detail?* I was going to burst. I had to remember to breathe, breathe, breathe.

She continued with her examination. Jacklyn was still on her side on the examination table. Then, with one hand on Jacklyn's back, the doctor slowly turned to us and stated in a whisper of a voice, "You both have done a noble job, a very noble effort as her parents, but it's time to discontinue the brace."

I was blindsided. I thought, *After all these years and discomfort, we* ***had*** *to continue to control this curve. Just like that, we're done? Why were we totally abandoning its use?*

Karl and the physiatrist left me to dress Jacklyn as they walked down the long hallway. Their discussion was barely audible to me. As we exited the professional/office building, Karl turned to me, saying, "She feels nothing more can be done." Looking at him, I could tell by his wrinkled brow that he, too, was uncomfortable. "The doctor said, 'Why put more stress on Jacklyn? Right now, she has a 90-degree curve.'" All I could think was that this was the beginning of the end. I was now worried that future changes were going to be made because we had reached the end of what the medical community can offer her. Lately, Jacklyn had hated when I put the brace on her. So, in an odd way, I was glad this would be one less piece of equipment—especially one that was so uncomfortable.

As we started our trip home, I repeated, "She is going to be fine. This will pass. She will be fine."

Karl nodded, "Yes, let's hope so."

Karl is grounded, so logical, whereas I'm not. The more I thought she would be fine, the more I was in denial—an inner dialogue that I instinctively welcomed. Here I go again: My "denial zone" helped free my emotions to refocus myself on other issues, giving me false peace. It was a safe place so my mind could rest. It soothed me. This "selective hearing" defense was an added benefit. It protected me from the punches—it was my shield, my armor. I liked this "zone," this sheltered place and have used it often—far *too* often these past nine and one-half years. I was hiding in that space, sometimes peeking out.

Running for the train to start another workweek, I tried to put aside the chilling fact that, on that day, Jacklyn did not have to wear her brace for the first time in years. No more fussing to show her unhappiness, no more sweating during the summer, no more, no more! She was free. I felt liberated just knowing she was comfortable, but, at the same time, the worry that I had now was scaring me to a different level.

Even my "denial zone" was not hiding or soothing. It was right up in my face, clear, palpable. I struggled to escape those thoughts and think about her upcoming tenth birthday. My mind was fighting an internal battle; it controlled everything I did and said. It was exhausting, draining, depleting everything within me. I forced myself, digging down deep with every bit of strength, to stop thinking that removal of her body brace might be the beginning of the end.

Instead, I pushed myself to start planning a birthday party. This was so contrary to the awful feeling I kept inside that I thought she would never make it to ten years old—that "magic number" day. A milestone that many doctors predicted she would not accomplish since their expectation of her living just a few years. I never imagined she would reach her tenth birthday celebration.

Instead of eating with co-workers in our lunchroom, I felt that a walk would clear my mind. Jamaica Avenue, the main hub of the Long Island Railroad, on that August day was hot and noisy with the sounds of trains, cars, and pedestrians rushing to their destinations. The smells of different ethnic foods permeated each passing block.

After strolling a few blocks, I came upon a storefront filled with crocheted baby items. I walked in to admire the handiwork and found it filled with little handmade dresses, blankets, hats, sweaters, and other accessories.

A young, dark-haired woman approached me. She said, "*Como puedo ayudarle?*" I guessed she was asking me in Spanish if I needed help. Before I could respond, I envisioned Jacklyn in a pure white crocheted dress like one that was on display. But all these dresses were for babies and toddlers, not a ten-year-old girl.

The sales lady realized I didn't understand Spanish and then continued in English. Choking to get my words out, I explained that my daughter would be ten years old soon but that she is a special child. She had reached only a one-month level. I wanted a special dress for her big day. I showed her a picture of Jacklyn, and then she showed me a photo of her two little girls. At that moment, I wasn't just a customer, and she wasn't just a saleswoman. Sharing that common bond of motherhood, that unconditional love for our children, I felt a connection to her. This stranger, while still holding Jacklyn's photo, looked into my eyes, reached across the counter, held my hand, and then promised to fulfill the uncommon request.

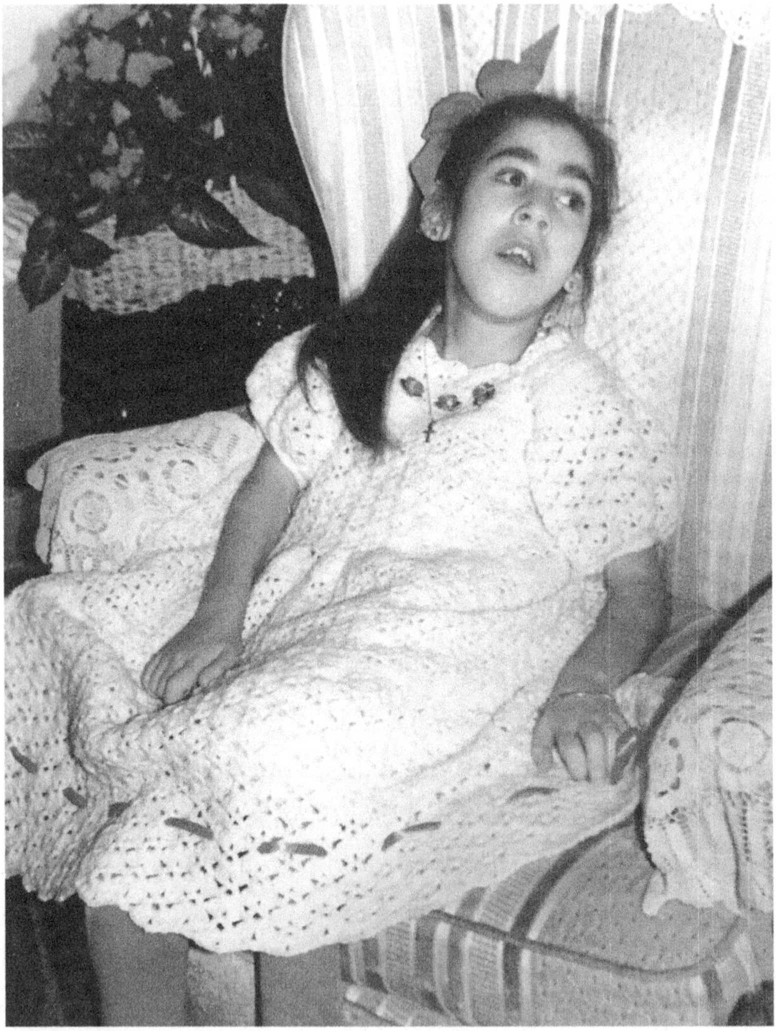

She assured me that a larger dress for a young girl could be made in approximately two weeks. I just had to supply the measurements.

I was ecstatic. I walked back to my office happily humming the *Sesame Street* theme tune "Sunny Day." I passed all the crowds, crying children, cars, trucks, and street odors as if they were invisible to my senses, almost bouncing with every step. Jacklyn would be glowing for her tenth birthday in this creation.

Walking quickly to get back to work, I noticed a fabric store on the next block, and my imagination started exploding with ideas. Thread a pink ribbon through the open spaces, and then match it up with pink tights and a hair bow, *plus* pink stick-on earrings for the special occasion. The finishing touch would be adorning the top part of the dress with matching little rosebuds. I would have loved to make her a dress like my mother often did for me when I was growing up, but I didn't have the talent. I may not have been making it with my own hands, but it would be created with love from my heart.

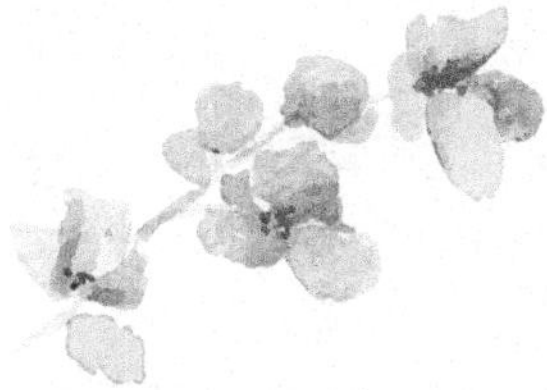

"The best and most beautiful things in the world cannot be seen or even touched—they must be felt with the heart."

—Helen Keller

Every Child Should Fly

It was a beautiful day, so I was heading down Nassau Blvd. It's just one of many times I'd taken Jacklyn to our local park during the last nine years. The only piece of equipment we could use is the swing. The closer I got to the park, the more I realized that I couldn't do this much longer, and I was frustrated. She has gotten too heavy, and I was fearful that I might drop her. I was strained beyond my physical boundaries. I'd known this for some time. Trying to hold onto and swing an almost ten-year-old young girl while she was in my lap was insane.

As I rolled her into the park entrance, the pain stung and bit at me. It had never gotten any better. Just seeing the other mothers with their healthy children who were riding, climbing, and swinging without a care—even if they fell and bruised their knees—has crippled me and left me alone. No one has *ever* approached us—not even a warm "hello." I would have given up everything to have Jacklyn bruise her knee and be part of this playground's bruised-knee gang. I felt angry but couldn't direct my fury at anyone there. I was angry at the world—a misplaced rage that ate at me and burned a hole in my chest, heart, and soul.

I desperately tried to think of the positive, turning away so as not to look in their direction. Somehow, I managed to block everyone at the park out of my senses. I wanted to be the only two people in the park, the only two people who matter. After all these years, it still created an inferno that travels within, all consuming, especially when stares come our way. The slightest glance, even an innocent one, will ignite the flame. Was this jealousy that I was feeling? Was I jealous of all the other mothers? Was I going insane?

I caressed Jacklyn's cheek and told her she will be flying on a swing again soon. Feeling her baby-soft face soothed me. Her warm cheeks comforted and calmed me. If she was happy, my feelings wouldn't count. Quickly, I veered off onto the left pathway, where there were fewer families and no other children using the swings. Still focusing, I concentrated on how she had enjoyed the trip to the park and hearing the cars and trucks that drive by, birds chirping, and the voices of other children. Yes, she enjoyed smelling the fresh-cut grass, rolling over the bumps and the uneven pavement, too. I was thankful for the little and big bumps that jiggle her and make her happy and sometimes produce a smile. I didn't want to give any of this up. I'm her protector, her advocate. How could I take away this childhood rite of passage when she had so little?

I calculated the least number of steps back to the swing's thin, black rubber seat, readjusted her chair closer, and then locked the brakes. Recalling instructions that I'd received on the proper way to lift, I bent my knees while keeping my back straight. When I began picking her up, she started to stiffen and hyperextend her body. I struggled in pain and didn't give a damn which back, leg, or neck muscles I needed to use to get her into the seat.

Her weight on my legs was cutting off my circulation. They were starting to feel numb. Tingling! I pushed a few times, but the swing was too low to the ground to get much movement. The sensation of flying like a bird with the wind that freely brushed her hair and face was now almost nonexistent. I stopped, exhausted, my hands aching from the tight pressure that leaves marks, almost breaking the skin. I waited to regain some feeling in my legs before lifting and placing her into the wheelchair. My legs were still wobbly but slowly regaining strength.

She looked up, toward the noise the other children were making, at the nearby slide and sand pit. My heart sank. I was losing it and had to leave the play area, pushing her past the happy children. My emotions were running high. *Was this another ending? Eating food by mouth—gone! Back brace—gone! Swing—gone!* This time I walked back home, taking the quiet streets, avoiding the noisy boulevard.

I slowly pushed the wheelchair, telling Jacklyn, "I'm going to fix this problem." Within a few blocks, she fell asleep. She looked so peaceful, innocent. With each bump in the pavement, I mentally recalled what she had lost, what she had been deprived of in life. A solution to this had to be found *now*!

The next day, after searching the telephone directory, I listed a few key numbers. I was going to call as many people as possible to get Jacklyn an appropriate swing. The first call redirected me to another department. I crossed off the first number and then dialed the second. I was put on hold and then disconnected. I redialed and was put on hold again. I was starting to get annoyed, but I held my temper. I'd gone through this with government bureaucracy and insurance, so it was nothing new. Fight, fight, fight—at times I felt I'd won if all I did was get my point across.

Eventually a pleasant voice gave me a direct number and wished me luck. I knew what was needed because I'd noticed this curved, shaped seat at a playground at one of the hospitals we visited and at United Cerebral Palsy of Nassau in Roosevelt, Long Island. If they could have a handicap swing, so could our local park. I dialed the direct number.

A week after my phone calls, we were sitting at the kitchen table, having lunch. The phone rang, and I picked it up on the second ring. "Yes—sure, I'll make an appointment." I turned to Karl, and I was going to burst. Explode! I couldn't believe what I'd heard. Was I dreaming?

"Karl, they are very willing to accommodate the swing. They want to meet with me, but first I'll have to research the exact piece of equipment." The next phase of playground renovation was scheduled for completion mid-October of that year. The parks department had it within their budget and would acquire and install the new handicap equipment. It was perfect timing.

The joy of knowing this project I'd pursued could bring a smile to not only Jacklyn but to other special children gave me an emotional high. It had been a long time since I'd bubbled inside with genuine happiness. This taste of victory was sweet—gloriously sweet!—knocking down the negativity that surrounded me. Karl couldn't contain himself, either. We hugged and yelled. He looked at me differently, with a look of pride I couldn't explain.

With my help, any child, regardless of ability, would soon enjoy our playground. I was sure that, when other mothers heard, they would come visit. Maybe meet for playdates. We can all be different together.

Being an advocate and winning for once lightened my heart. I started calling my family and friends with the news. It felt good, really good! *Jacklyn will be flying like a bird again.* Yes, it's scheduled to be installed right after her eleventh birthday.

New York State and Medically Fragile Children

Jacklyn might die today. That was the only thought in my mind as I looked out the passenger-side window. We were heading to the emergency room yet again. I was trembling, shaking so hard that I broke out in a sweat—feeling every pore try to extinguish the fire on my skin. I couldn't control my quivering. I tried, by wrapping my arms around my body, squeezing tightly, but had little luck. All I could do was bite my lip and wait until my body was exhausted from the episode. I should have been accustomed to this physical reaction, but I was not. How could I possibly get accustomed to the fact that my child might die today? Within minutes, life could change.

Half an hour before, I'd come home to the phone ringing. I heard Karl saying, "Hello. I understand. Okay—we will leave now." He rushed past me. "Leave your coat on; that was

Ferncliff, and they said Jacklyn is having trouble breathing." As we drove to the hospital, I knew what Karl was imagining.

Arriving at the emergency room, we ran into the hospital, leaving the car halfway on the sidewalk and halfway on the road. Karl was being asked questions, and I could hear him answer, "Last year at the children's hospital, a swallow study determined that fluid was entering her lungs, so she received a gastric feeding tube."

Everyone was rushing around us. I sat on her bed and tucked the blanket across her chest, trying to provide extra warmth over the thin hospital gown. I whispered, "Don't be scared. Mommy and Daddy are here," as I stroked her face. I got to hold her hand for a brief few minutes before they whisked her away for tests. Trying to follow, I was told to wait. As I watched the hospital staff roll her down the polished-gray long corridor floor, part of me was still attached—the invisible part that can never be broken.

I didn't know how much time had passed, but eventually the emergency room doctor returned to us. He stated, "She needs a cuffed tracheotomy." Karl and I looked at each other with puzzled expressions and then turned to the doctor. He started to go into detail.

Stunned, I felt like I was melting into a puddle while trying to listen to the physician's clarification. Karl had to slowly explain the findings to me more than once. "Look at me. Listen to me carefully. She keeps getting pneumonia. She needs this procedure, or the fluids entering her lungs will eventually kill her."

I started to shake and tremble again. "Are you saying that they are going to put a hole in her throat?" I'd seen this on other, much older, patients. But, never in my wildest dreams, could I have imagined this would be done to my daughter.

Karl then took my hand. "Sit down and listen closely. A cuffed tracheotomy means there will be a small balloon inside the trach that we must inflate on a schedule. This will help prevent saliva from entering her lungs."

When you look at Jacklyn's face, she is beautiful: silky, thick auburn hair, milky-white skin, full eyebrows, and big brown eyes. This provided a mask for me to hide behind. It was an image in which nothing was wrong, a photo to give to family and friends of my pretty child. Her problems could remain my own secret. I didn't notice the drool on her chin, her unresponsive blank stares, the wheelchair, the leg braces, the grimace from a seizure. No, I didn't notice all of those because I had that one picture that didn't show her flaws, seeing her as my heart sees her, not my eyes. Capturing that one picture enabled me to hide behind it when I needed shelter. It might take 100 attempts to secure that one perfect photo, but that was the one I carried in my heart. It was the one I proudly showed when I wasn't looking for pity or whispers behind my back. It was the one I used to hide behind when I didn't want her to be different.

After the surgery, I would not be able to hide her disabilities like before. I wouldn't be able to continue the charade. *When people glanced, how would I deal with my embarrassment? I won't be able to conceal it. But I shouldn't hide; my feelings are not important.*

They are a miniscule dot, a speck not worthy of mention. If she has the surgery, I'll stand by her, endure the children's gawking, absorb what she cannot see and love her more—if that was even humanly possible. I would do it in a heartbeat. But, would it be painless and help her? So far, my doubts were strong and persistent.

Another surgery? How could I agree to this one? This would be another major change within one year, and we were told the tracheotomy would then classify her as medically fragile. I was starting to count, mentally list all the changes: no more brace, feeding through a tube in her stomach, and now a tube will be placed in her throat. They were adding up, and all heading in the wrong direction.

I recalled years ago, when I'd seen some forms of happiness—that slight smile, happy grunt, those little signs that meant the world to me. That gave me the desire and hope for better days. They were so limited, infrequent, and yet I worshiped any good moments she could experience.

As I watched the fading changes with each passing year and now possibly again, it created a numbness that I cannot describe because there are no words that could adequately explain this level of sorrowfulness. I couldn't bear to hurt her anymore. Her quality of life was declining. I could see and feel the difference. It ate at me. Ripped at me. I had been worrying for a long time that the doctors were grasping at straws. She was only ten and a half years old and had been through so many surgical procedures—more than most adults in their lifetime. Plus, if she had this surgery, she would not be able to return to Ferncliff Manor, because they were not qualified to handle tracheotomy care—an enormous setback!

What would happen if we did nothing? Her saliva would continue to enter her lungs and shorten her life span. Have we been selfish? Have all these surgeries been for her or for us?

The next day we returned to the hospital with a mandatory appointment to speak to a gentleman from the hospital's ethical department. I didn't know what to expect as we sat down at a long beige table in a private conference room. I was uncomfortable, my leg restlessly shaking under the table to release the tension. I sensed this was a room where people were brought to discuss awful decisions.

As he opened the door, my leg was shaking more vigorously. He strolled into the room, introduced himself, and stated, "We are here today to discuss your daughter Jacklyn, who is a minor child." I watched as he shuffled around a stack of folders, thinking, *How many other families will he be speaking to today? How many other lives will he touch?*

He continued, "The advised new procedure would help prevent the reoccurrence of her pneumonia and is not considered extraordinary measures for her survival." Studying him and trying to comprehend the full purpose of this meeting, he reminded me of a teacher in a classroom, following a curriculum with his open textbook. The more he spoke, the more I detected a legal hospital obligation. He strongly emphasized she was a minor and couldn't communicate her wishes; therefore, hospital representation was necessary.

Exhaling, I was aware that the state had to protect those who cannot protect themselves. But this was different. I blocked him out, watching his mouth moving but not hearing any words. I shut him off completely after he mentioned that "I see that Jacklyn has a DNR. You know they aren't usually necessary in cases involving children. Young children have strong hearts. They don't normally have heart attacks that require resuscitation." I was aware of her DNR (Do Not Resuscitate). Steam was rising from my neck and face. *Damn it, why did he even mention that? I'm not stupid. I know that the elderly or terminally ill routinely have family members sign off on "do not resuscitate" orders. This meeting is making me sick to my stomach, and I want to get up and leave the room. Doesn't he realize he is talking about my daughter, my child, my baby?*

I started to gaze off, staring at a large picture of flowers on the wall behind him—shutting down all my senses to block out anything else he had to say. *How dare the hospital put us through this! How dare they give us more pressure and make us feel incompetent. We have enough to worry about. He is wasting our time. Does he think we are unfit to make the best decision for our child?*

Waiting for him to finish speaking and move onto the next family, the next folder, I reconnected only after hearing him state again that "it's not considered extraordinary measures." So, he is informing us that this is a standard procedure and yes, she probably will not die from heart failure. Could something else go wrong? If she survives, she ends up with a hole in her throat that *might* fix her problem—but for how much longer? And, he doesn't mention where the facility will be located that can manage all her medical necessities to survive.

All I could think was, *I don't want her to die. I don't want her to suffer. I don't have total trust in medical opinions anymore. I don't want the state or court to intervene.* Over and over, those thoughts repeated. These healthcare providers are invested in her care; they don't want to fail. They are so focused that they lose sight of the quality of life. Do they love her like we do? Do they understand her like we do? Can they read into every wrinkled brow, hand gesture, sound, twitch, grimace, or stare? I couldn't listen to him go on and on about what the hospital thought was good for our daughter. It was just another temporary fix in a long chain of their temporary fixes.

Leaving the room upon conclusion of the meeting, I turned to Karl: "No. Leave her alone. Enough is enough. We're tormenting her."

Karl nodded. He told me to separate my feelings, to remove them from the equation and focus on what is best for her now. "Calm down and think. The hospital's representative made it clear and is waiting for us to schedule the surgery. We don't have the energy or resources to fight and change opinions."

I was thinking crazy thoughts as I walked down the hallway. How could I have said that to Karl? How could I even consider not doing more surgery? I should want to do everything in the world possible to help my child—to keep her alive. I should travel to the ends of the Earth to save her. I was ashamed: *What kind of an awful monster, hideous mother have I turned into? I shouldn't think twice about this, yet I am.*

I had dreadful thoughts of people saying we were unfit parents if they learned that we didn't do what the hospital suggested. Lord knows what the hospital would do or say if we didn't comply. Would it be true that I'm an unfit mother? Or was my love for her so deep, so profound, that I can't be part of her suffering anymore? If she has another surgery and goes through more pain and distress and still gets worse, then it's on my conscience. I used to believe that doctors were gods who fixed everything. No, they are not. I'd be damned with either decision.

Looking for my approval, Karl said, "Please. Let me handle this. We have no choice." I continued to think this procedure should not be done.

Passing the small chapel, I went in and sat alone in one of the pews. Karl continued to the surgical department to arrange the date. As I sat, the day's events and mounting pressures were slowly replaying and crashing down around me. I was surrounded; the chapel's wooden wall paneling and wooden pews were sealing and confining me. I was in a box with no way to escape, buried, suffocating—cornered by the lack of options. *What did I do to create this mess? How did I get to this horrific place in my life? What sins have I committed?* I wished I knew. Nevertheless, it had to be my fault. There was a drive within me to repair what I had broken, to make things better.

The guilt I was holding inside was erupting again—an ugly monster emerging from the deepest portion of my mind. I needed to direct my anger, release the torment inside on some-one or something. I couldn't rid myself of the guilt that, since

I had carried Jacklyn, *I* had most likely caused her problems. It was something *I* did. Rocking back and forth, I tried to soothe myself as I rehashed my mental list of probable causes.

What did I do? What could it be? Eating too many tuna platters while I was pregnant? I should have known about the mercury in fish. It could have been the toxic droplet that fell on the floor from a broken thermometer. I was just a child, far too young to even realize touching the silver mercury could harm me—that it was a very dangerous substance. Also, I'd walked in and out of the house when Jacklyn's nursery was being painted—the paint fumes? Or was it the few glasses of wine I had before I found out I was pregnant? Plus, after her birth, I took her to the pediatrician's office for her DPT immunization. Years later the local news criticized this inoculation as a problem. It could be any of those or all of them.

I felt myself still rocking, but slower than before, as I tried to figure which was the likely culprit.

My back was stiff. My arms crossed and wrapped around my shoulders as I continued to rock. It neither relaxed nor lessened my racing mind. The aching stiffness had traveled from my back into my shoulders. The tension buildup in my shoulders soon traveled to my neck. The physical pain still didn't compare; how much greater can it grow to equal my mental pain?

At that point, my rocking had stopped, but the guilt shifted onto a different level. I wished I could stop thinking and shut my brain off, stop it from going from one awful moment to another. I was at the mercy of this evil seed that had been planted inside my brain—that grows and sprouts up whenever it wants control. I wanted to dig out the roots, every piece, and rid my mind of these feelings that were counterproductive, placing me into that deep dark hole. *I'm pathetic!*

Still more issues materialized. Now, it was the guilt of possibly not making all the correct medical decisions. I had tried to research every procedure and any possible path that could have produced the best outcome. Could there have been just one thing done differently that would have made a vast difference? Did we leave a stone unturned? Not gone to that one doctor who had the right treatment plan? That one recommendation from a friend that I didn't follow up on? I think not, but there was that one remote chance, that one single instance that would always leave a doubt that ate at me, poisoned, infected me, spread, and became all consuming.

Exhausted physically and mentally, my hands covered my face as I leaned over into my lap. I prayed for direction, a clear path. Sitting in the pew, moaning, I looked up, staring at Mother Mary near the altar. Her face was glowing bright from the overhead lights, peaceful and serene. I asked her to help me. To guide me. To save Jacklyn. Stop her reoccurring pneumonia. *Hail Mary, full of grace . . .*

The next day Jacklyn was having the operation while we anxiously paced in the surgical waiting room. The small area was almost empty except for one older man sitting quietly in the corner, staring at the floor. Karl and I were barely paying attention to the news report coming from the television mounted on the wall behind us. I turned and asked Karl, "What if she still gets pneumonia?"

Before he could utter a word, the doctor, still in his operating-room scrubs, slowly approached us. I stared at his face and then his eyes to get some sense that she had made it. I couldn't detect any emotion. I stood, my body getting rigid. I could hear my heart pounding. I stood stiff, waiting for the next blow. Would he say, "I'm sorry, Mr. and Mrs. Messina"? If he started off with those words, I'd know that my child died today.

He looked tired and briefly paused, interrupted by a co-worker. Why did he have to stop and speak to him? Why didn't this co-worker wait until he spoke to us first? After finishing the conversation, he greeted us. As I leaned against Karl, he said that the surgery went as expected and that we could go to her room and wait.

Exhaling, I released my clenched fists. I wanted to run and catch the next elevator, but my legs felt like rubber. Weaving in and out, we headed to her room, passing all the beeping machines and various carts along the hallway. We walked in, and the hospital bed, with its crisp, tightly folded linen, was ready for its next guest.

It wasn't long before the attendant arrived with Jacklyn. She was still unconscious as I focused on the bandage covering her neck. Two nurses entered. The taller, more mature woman handed us a booklet, while a much younger nurse followed her commands and hooked Jacklyn up to various machines. She said, "Please read the maintenance book. It's important. I'll be back later."

Reading the instructions on tracheostomy and cuff care, I felt my child wasn't going to tolerate it well. I knew from that moment that I, too, would have a problem. I couldn't remove the plastic tube from her throat to clean and replace it. I couldn't handle the maintenance or the suctioning out any mucus. I was desperately trying to stay strong, but I couldn't. I was failing. I was weak.

Waiting for her to fully recover from the anesthesia, I was withdrawn, distant. Her limp hand was warm. I tenderly kissed it. My eyes closed as I dozed off. I was running, faster and faster. Looking behind, everyone was staring and pointing at me. I ran down the steps, passing dozens of mothers holding their children, and found myself at the lobby door. I hesitated to exit, and then, I abruptly dashed to my car.

"Did you fall asleep?" Karl was calling me. "Did you fall asleep?"

Opening my eyes, I looked at him and said, "Yes."

For years, I had tried to treat her to a somewhat normal existence, but all of it was hitting me so hard now: *She isn't normal. No, she isn't.* Just giving her a bath or cooling off in a pool could be devastating. Water could flood her lungs through the tube, drowning her. Had we made the right decision? This surgery, this time? Should we have been firm, if possible, and done nothing? Placed her in God's hands? *Oh, how I wish I could trade places with her. I wish it were me. What do I have to negotiate with? What could I offer in trade—my eyes, my legs, my voice, my soul? Yes, if I could, I would trade my soul to help my innocent child.*

She woke up, coughing up mucus through the tracheotomy tube. I was surprised and almost paralyzed with fear. Karl shouted, "Go to the nurse's station to get help." I watched as Jacklyn's primary care nurse quickly removed the thick substance. All I could do was hold Jacklyn's hand as I wiped away my tears. I found it extremely difficult to look at the surgery site. Karl was much stronger—he always was. She continued to remove the remaining mucus as Karl observed.

After the crisis passed, we resumed reading the maintenance instructions. I turned to him and shook my head. "I can't do this. I can't. Please, please no."

Karl replied, "It's okay. I can handle it until you're ready."

"I don't know if I'll ever be ready," I said as I looked down to the floor and held my head.

The nurse would be coming back later. She had to be convinced that one of us could handle this procedure as well as emergency insertion, just in case the tube falls out. She'd already given us a heads-up that, no matter what facility we find to replace Ferncliff Manor, someone in our home must be capable. Otherwise, Jacklyn would never be released for home visits. For now, I had to accept the fact that Karl would have to perform the trach maintenance. I couldn't think. I couldn't keep up. Just an endless string of worries, day after day. I'm drained. *God, are you testing me beyond my limits?*

Cuff Care

1. Inflate when sleeping
2. Can deflate when on her side
3. Inflate when feeding and keep for one hour after

4. Deflate x hours a day for a total of 3 hours
   (Space out for 1 hour 3 x a day.)
5. Approx. 2 cc air for cuff.
   (Do not make full—should be soft)

Tracheostomy Care

1. Remove cannula
2. Mix ½ saline and ½ peroxide
3. Dip Q-tips into above
4. Clean area
5. Place inner cannula into solution. Rinse/soak cannula.
6. Use clear water or saline to go over area after using solution of ½ saline and ½ peroxide. Dry cannula in and out.
7. Suction out all mucus
8. Dry area (Q-tips and gauze cloths) around stoma and apply cream
9. Replace cannula

The hospital's Patient Advocate caught me as I re-entered Jacklyn's room the following morning. Jacklyn was now classified *medically fragile* by the state of New York. The Patient Advocate explained that we had to find a facility that can handle her tracheostomy care, a residence that provides 24-hour professional nursing. Ferncliff was not on the list of facilities providing that service. We'd grown attached to and trusted the Ferncliff staff, making it more difficult to say goodbye.

Shaking my head, I promised to make an appointment with her. We were treading in new, uncharted waters. The definition of an "advocate" is a person who speaks or writes in support. I hoped so. We would see!

Days passed, and I found myself sitting in the hospital office of our Patient Advocate. Jacklyn had stabilized, and the advocate now wanted us to quickly move her into a new rehabilitation facility. She handed me a list of homes to visit that were options. I noticed that few handle trach patients. Her title now bewildered me. How was this *advocacy*?

The first and second facility we visited were close to home. Each location gave us the same impression. There was an eerie stillness as I walked the hallways until a loud yell from one of the patients would break the silence. The smell of urine was present most of the time. The patients were between fifty and ninety years old, and, for the most part, these were geriatric nursing homes! I didn't notice cheerful expressions on any of the staff. Jacklyn would have been the only child at each location, with no activities or school for her age bracket, no children for Jacklyn to hear, removing her only sense of enjoyment. I would *never* allow this placement. A geriatric nursing home is not a place for my child. How could the "advocate" even list these as a possibility? It's all about dollars and cents.

Late in the afternoon, I returned to the Patient Advocate's small office and sat in the vacant chair next to a huge pile of folders. Tension was rising between us because she wanted us out of the hospital. If I bowed down and appeased her, then

I'd have failed as my daughter's advocate and protector. Hell, there would be nothing left!

She commented, "Jacklyn is ready to be transferred tomorrow. Which facility did you pick?" At the same time, she pushed the consent release forms for me to sign in my direction.

I paused to control my temper as I held the list tightly in my hand. The friction was mounting as I looked at her while she was casually tending to her paperwork. She inquired again. Slamming down the useless list on her desk, I yelled that it would be "over my dead body" if my daughter was placed in any of those facilities. I glared at her while getting up and, in a guttural tone, repeated, "Over my dead body."

Avoiding my piercing stare, she huffed and shook her head while gazing downward. I walked out of her office, leaving the crumpled, unsigned hospital paperwork tossed onto her desk.

After that day, I became oblivious to the passage of time, concentrating all my efforts in one direction. I was unable to eat or sleep in search of a placement for Jacklyn—what I started calling "a piece of heaven on Earth." There were no acceptable institutions to be found on Long Island. We would have to travel more than 120 miles and possibly into another state. I've learned that the more medically complicated a person is, it creates much more difficulty in finding a facility close to home. The odds are even more remote for placing a child. And, a child with a tracheostomy—hell, it would be easier finding a needle in a haystack.

Taking out my frustrations on anyone and everyone who would listen to me, I vented my rage to neighbors, hospital personnel, and family members—all while messages from the Patient Advocate continued to arrive. This didn't make any sense to me! Jacklyn and other children like her should be placed close to their home in order for parents to make *all* those important medical decisions. Why are they placed *far* from home and parents, grandparents, siblings? Why are other states taking our children, when we could create jobs and give them services right here? More insanity! Am I the only person who sees this is clearly wrong?

All during this same period, Karl and I both had our eyes and ears open to other options closer to home. Through networking, we found that the construction of a group home for medically fragile children near to us was under consideration.

The List! We're on The List! I thought. We put Jacklyn's name on a list of possible candidates for this proposed local group home. I had to be patient. Every day, I wondered if that would be the day that we'd get the call that our eleven-year-old daughter had been picked out of what I was told was 600 waiting children labeled by the state as "medically fragile." Only six would be chosen if the capital budget got passed. I needed to have hope—hope that she would be close by and not more than 120 miles away.

I needed to have hope that she would not be placed out of state or in a geriatric-oriented nursing home. How could our government representatives *not* pass this and even give additional funding to support so many families like us? This would open a door to keeping our family together. With Jacklyn's bouts of pneumonia, a feeding tube in her stomach, a tracheostomy, and the fact that she was not seizure free, legislators had to realize she needs round-the-clock, skilled care. If I could go to Albany and speak to our lawmakers, I would simply say, "How would *you* feel if *you* were separated by a great distance from your blind child who cannot speak a single word?"

For too long, these children and young adults had been *invisible* to the rest of society. Yet, my Jacklyn is not invisible! No, not invisible to me. I can sense her happy moments. I can tell if her braces are pinching when no one else notices. I can sense when she has a temperature. There is a mystical, magical, spiritual connection, a bond that cannot be broken. I *feel* it—no words are needed. Her big brown eyes often search in the direction of a familiar sound or a bright overhead light. I love to comb her thick, silky auburn hair. No, she is not *invisible* to me.

It will pass. It will pass, I repeated as a daily mantra. *Jacklyn will be chosen for this facility, and, at last, I'll be at peace,* I would say to myself to try to stop my insides from quivering. My thoughts dwelled on the fact her mental capacity was only that of a one-month-old. It haunted me and kept me on constant alert, attentive to her needs, like a mother with a newborn. She would be my "Forever Baby." *It will pass. It will pass.* I needed to rest my fears, but the quivering continued, and it hurt. My insides hurt. I was afraid for her and for us as a family. She simply couldn't be placed hours from us. We were in limbo. It was as if nobody could see us. It was as if no one *wanted* to notice.

It was an early Saturday morning, and I'd just returned from shopping with my food list in my hand of neatly crossed-off items. This list was short, but it gave me a sense of control. Yes, control of what was picked and what was bypassed. It reminded me in an odd way that this must be what the legislators were doing. They were picking which children and young adults would be at the top of the list of those in need of 24-hour care. Money shouldn't have been an issue, yet I was not so naïve to be unaware that, just as in purchasing items off the food shelves, the lower-priced item is preferred when you're on a budget. This was insane! How could our representatives put a price tag on this? *It will pass. It will pass,* I whispered to myself and left the supermarket.

Karl came out to meet me and helped unload the car. He must have been waiting at the door for my return. I glanced at his face. His blue eyes were red. Without hesitation, he took my hand and said, "I just got the call. The budget failed."

Almost falling to my knees, I couldn't even cry. I have nothing more left. "How could this be?" I repeat. Another dashed dream. I couldn't think straight as I crumpled up the grocery list and threw it to the ground. We entered the house, and there was silence—the empty kind of silence that I'd lived through far too often. The silence that comes with a broken heart, a scattered dream, the lonely isolation. The silence that comes with being different.

The state bureaucrats and legislators had cut funding, so there would not be a place on Long Island for any "medically fragile" children this year. The budget cuts halted Jacklyn's access as well as that of a few other children to live near their families. Again, it was all about dollars and cents. Devastated, I couldn't come to grips with the callous fact Jacklyn was just another number, just a statistic. Not only were we different as a family, we were *forgotten* by government and society. She had become invisible. I had to fight to make her visible because she is *real*—our problems were *real*, and they ripped at the family core and destroyed the basic family unit.

This was another battle, a life-or-death crusade. I considered going to Washington, DC, with Jacklyn. They had to see who was being affected by their decisions. Our representatives need to understand the urgency. But how? How the hell could I prove my point? It didn't take me long to accept that my idea would not be practical. It was a fantasy. Who was I kidding? I would need a team of skilled helpers to attempt such a trip.

A few days passed, and I was still numb—I had no feelings. I was devoid of any emotion. I was oblivious to the sights and sounds around me. I was dead inside, yet I was still breathing. I'd been there before, in that state of abandonment, but this time, it was more critical. We didn't have another plan. There wasn't another "list." There was little hope, few, if any, choices close to home for our special child.

I was mad, outraged. I started writing a letter but hadn't decided who I should send it to. Maybe the entire country should read this and reconsider how they treat their handicapped children. I wanted to challenge our government to create a law that would allow our special children to stay close to home.

To: ?
Subject: Jacklyn's Journey

Today's advanced technology has given our young medically fragile population a greater chance of survival, but our government has dismissed or ignored the simple fact of a proper facility to care for these delicate charges. I am thankful for all the advanced technology for prolonging my child's life, but how shortsighted our elected officials have become in creating suitable housing for these children as they age. People with disabilities already have limited choices. They are our vulnerable population. Why are they being restricted as to where they should be allowed to call home?

Would government and state officials fund and build a bridge from a city that leads nowhere? Would they drop off travelers in the middle of a vast wasteland? I think NOT! Are these children any less human when they reach a certain age—do they just become transparent and dismissed from the minds of our elected officials? Do our lawmakers hope that they will fade out behind closed doors and out of the public eye?

Signed: Broken-Hearted Mother

St. Mary's

Jacklyn's music box was playing "Raindrops Keep Fallin' on My Head" while I was unpacking her clothing. It was almost evening, and we were at St. Mary's Hospital for Children in Bayside, Queens.

It had all started one week ago. A prayer had been answered when Jacklyn's trusted physiatrist informed us about St. Mary's. It was located less than thirty minutes from our home. She explained that they had rehab programs for children. It was considered a temporary site, but if we actively looked for a long-term home, we would not be harassed and forced out. I trusted her opinion and made plans for us to tour the facility.

Arriving late in the afternoon, we entered the building, walking past a statue of the Blessed Mother and a fresh flower bed. I picked up a pamphlet, and we both started reading how St. Mary's president had dedicated himself to improving the health and quality of life for children with special needs and their families. He'd created programs when none existed.

Yet, with so many prior disappointments, I turned to Karl and said, "I'm not getting my hopes up."

As we turned to walk down the hallway, a man with a big smile, small in stature with salt-and-pepper hair, started to approach us. You could feel his warm personality projecting with his extended handshake. He said, "You must be the Messinas. Welcome to St. Mary's Hospital for Children" and invited us to have dinner in the nearby cafeteria. He told the cashier not to charge us. Then he quickly looked at his watch, waved goodbye, and swiftly left, dashing down the corridor.

Karl and I were both surprised and a bit puzzled. We yelled "Thank you" to this gentleman, who'd already disappeared from our view, while we proceeded to the counter. The cafeteria was immaculate, and the jovial server in an oversized white apron filled our trays. Happy children's voices echoed throughout the facility. It was sweet music to our ears. The louder the reverberations, the more tranquil and secure I felt.

The hamburger and fries tasted like steak from a fine-dining restaurant. We looked at each other and smiled. I blurted out, "We can't be this lucky." Karl's contented expression echoed my feelings. Yes, he felt it, too. Soon after finishing our meal, we continued to review the pamphlet. Turning the page, we saw a picture of the man we'd just met. We realized that the gentleman who'd cheerfully greeted us was the president. Soon, I felt this rush, this feeling of acceptance that spread like a wave and filled all my senses. It was the first time I'd had dinner with my husband surrounded by the overwhelming impression of a safe environment for Jacklyn that was *not* far from our home.

Within minutes, our tour guide approached our table, introduced herself, and brought us to the different units within the building. A therapy room had a young therapist cheering on a small boy walking with crutches. So proud of himself, he offered up such an engaging smile. Across from them was another child draped over a large ball, and her therapist was gently moving the ball, almost bouncing it, as the child attempted to raise her head. I noticed a surprised expression as the therapist said, "Good job."

The play area had children, some in wheelchairs and others in tumble-form seating systems like the one Jacklyn was using. They were all seated in a circle. Music was playing, and one little girl's face reminded me of Jacklyn's when she heard music. Her eyes opened wide and turned toward the melody. Instantly, I pictured Jacklyn there in that room with the others.

Next, the classrooms we passed were filled with adaptive equipment and art supplies. Upon further inspection, I spotted assorted items for each level of ability. Each room, whether it was a therapy room, school classroom, or play area, had ample equipment. Room after room, I couldn't find anything that wouldn't stand up to any parent's close scrutiny. Another wave of calm and tranquility came over me. My inner fear began to subside, serenity overtaking and crushing my demons. Wherever I turned, I saw and heard joyful youngsters, even though they struggled with their disabilities. It was a clean, odor-free multicomplex with smiling staff who appeared knowledgeable and attentive to the children's needs. We went back to our tour guide's office, and, with my lap full of various pamphlets, a feeling of reassurance overcame me.

Our tour representative asked if we had any other questions, and then she gave us some privacy to discuss our decision. Karl and I just glanced at each other and smiled. I hadn't smiled that much in such a long time that my cheeks hurt.

"Karl, my cheek muscles are hurting! Who knew that would happen?"

While still grinning, too, he said, "I think we have found a temporary reprieve." We would now have the time to search for a permanent home that best suited Jacklyn and our family.

The decision was made, and we arranged to have Jacklyn transferred. Upon leaving the building, I could hear some staff members leading children in a song as they walked down the hallway. I thanked God for directing us here. I shuddered to think of what would have happened had I accepted any of the other, geriatric sites out of desperation. I was sick to my stomach recalling those facilities, where there was eerie stillness until a loud yell from one of the patients would echo throughout the hallways.

I visited daily to make sure all of Jacklyn's medical and daily living needs were being met satisfactorily. Daily hugs and kisses were on the top of my list, and I took advantage of every opportunity. After not seeing her for the entire day, I would feel exhilarated—as if I had just won the top prize at a carnival game—whenever I noticed a happy expression. I would occasionally catch the slightest of smiles, so very faint and brief. Lately, I had to wait longer to catch one of them. With each year that passed, they had become less frequent,

But also less frequent was my desire to mask my feelings. I knew my happily-ever-after had been broken beyond repair. I had to hold on to one factor. I could tell she was being treated well. Our good insurance coverage accepted this top-rated facility, and that took the additional stress from our plate. Lord knows what would have happened if we'd had to quit our jobs to move out of state to find her a qualified residence, losing our healthcare coverage. But that was another worry for another time, because, at that moment, I was back to being Jacklyn's mom—not just her caretaker. Karl and I had time to regain some of our strength, the respite we both desperately needed to get ready to fight the next battle.

I requested that the staff let Jacklyn's music box play at bedtime, so she knew it was time to go to sleep. I'd always made it an evening routine. This little wooden musical toy had a serene, soothing, and peaceful tune. It played "Raindrops Keep Fallin' on My Head," and I always tried to sing the lyrics that meant the most to me. It was a tribute to how we survived another day.

Music had always been important. Listening to any of her musical toys would remind me of prior summers. All those warm days when she was home, I had another routine. I would take advantage of the Mister Softee Ice Cream truck in a totally unusual way compared to most families. It frequently drove past our house, attracting children to purchase delicious treats. Whenever I would hear the truck's jingle off in the distance, I would rush to open as many windows as possible. The house soon filled with the melody while I yelled, "Jacklyn, listen to the big music box." She would perk up upon hearing the tune and turn toward the sound with wide eyes, crinkled-up nose, and a soft "grrrr." I wondered if it was the cheerful music or hearing all the children's voices that made her happy.

I recall looking out our big living room window and thinking how lucky those parents were to be able to enjoy such a simple thing with their children. *Do they realize what a gift they are experiencing?* They probably didn't give it a second thought. I would view the children walking hand in hand with their mother or father as they held their ice cream cones. Then, I would glance down at Jacklyn, propped up in her tumble-form molded chair as she turned toward the squeaky little voices of neighbors' children she would never get to know. I would see the droplets on her forehead coming from her hair, damp, sweating from the plastic that surrounded her.

They had their routine, and so did I. If this is what she enjoyed, as small as it may be, then so be it. My feelings didn't count. No, they didn't count at all. I continued with this ritual because Jacklyn enjoyed this even though it tore my insides to pieces. I watched all the other mothers and fathers with their young kids, walking, holding hands, eating ice cream. I often stared until they all disappeared down the block into fuzzy shadows and the ice cream truck drove so far away that I was unable to hear even a faint tune. My child didn't understand what was going on, and I wished I didn't, either.

That was the past, but now, Jacklyn was totally settled at St. Mary with her music boxes and a good supply of Disney and *Sesame Street* stories on tape. During the frequent drives to visit Jacklyn at St. Mary, I often noticed a young, long-haired petite woman walking to the facility. I didn't know if she'd traveled by train or bus, but nevertheless, her on-foot trek was more than a mile. I believed she was visiting someone, but I never saw her with any child. One day, I offered her a ride, but she declined. I hoped to meet her one day.

Jacklyn's first weekend visit at home from St. Mary was a tremendous undertaking. Watching Karl struggle to carry her up the front steps and then the interior steps to her room frightened me. I kept busy by unpacking the tracheostomy-care kit. This was the first time that we needed to handle it at home. The house was quiet except for the birds chirping in the tree in front of our house as Karl carried Jacklyn into her bedroom. The wheelchair couldn't clear the narrow doorway.

I stood outside her bedroom, leaning against the hallway wall, wishing I had more courage. Karl said, "Please go into the kitchen and prepare the saline-and-peroxide solution." Without delay, I poured the mixture while the gurgling and suctioning of mucus echoed throughout the quiet house. Heading toward her bedroom with the bowl of solution, I could hear this strange sound coming from her—an unfamiliar sound. Her small grunts now were sounds of air whisking through a plastic pipe, unrecognizable as a voice. Yet this was now her voice. The playful sounds that I had become used to were gone. Her form of communication had silenced forever—it had been taken, stolen from her small body. Destiny had now removed yet another piece of my child, and, with it, another piece of me, too. I knew she was upset. I could feel it.

Entering her bedroom, I wanted to console her, but I was frozen as I watched Karl place a plastic tube into the hole, removing the last bit of mucus. Placing the bowl down, I looked away. As I slowly brought my eyes upward, I saw a frightened expression on her face. She started to cough, her face turning red; then there was an absence of any sound—a cough with no sound. Again, another cough, and again no sound. Karl continued to follow the instruction sheet from the hospital.

All I could do was sit next to her, hold her hand, and say, "I'm sorry." I feel her pain, I sensed her fear. I'm broken, empty inside, and the only strength that I can draw upon is watching how my husband can handle yet another obstacle without me. I'm too weak. I cannot perform this task.

She had been moved to a different floor at St. Mary's Hospital because the cuffed trach was not preventing all secretions from entering her lungs. Yet, I focused on one thing: She was close to home, close to me. One weekend, my mom wanted to visit Jacklyn, so I picked her up and was looking forward to an enjoyable day together. I purchased a nature tape of birds singing and was excited to play it for Jacklyn. I knew she would enjoy the familiar warbling.

We arrived and took the elevator up to her new location in the Palliative Care Unit on the top floor. As we entered, I noticed the same young woman I'd seen on the road and wanted to introduce myself since we now had more of a connection. Both our children were on the same floor. Maybe if she got to know me, she would accept a ride the next time. I just needed to break the ice. Her back was facing me as I came within reach. She was holding her baby and appeared to be feeding the child. As my mom and I approached we froze. Peering over the woman's shoulder, we were both deeply shaken.

Her back still facing us, she didn't notice us. Gently taking my mother's arm, I guided her away, down the long hallway, toward Jacklyn's room. This young mother who I wanted to befriend was not feeding this child who was in her arms. No, this wasn't the case. The baby in her arms did not have a face. *My God—this baby didn't have a face!* At least not a recognizable, traditional face. All I could see was a gaping hole for what I thought was the baby's mouth and no noticeable nose or eyes. I have seen a great deal during years of hospital visits, but I was unprepared for this baby's deformity. Nevertheless, I felt a connection with this mother. We both loved our child unconditionally, no matter what challenges they sent our way.

As I continued to steer my mother toward Jacklyn's room, I looked to my right. Quickly, I placed my body to shield my mother's view of the room we were passing. I noticed a figure propped up in bed. This youngster's head was massive—maybe three times a normal size. Now, I felt like I was in a minefield, hoping to make it to safety. My peripheral vision saw two nurses attempting to reposition this young child. The wind was knocked out of me, and I was having trouble breathing as I continued to take my mother down the hallway.

We both sat in the side chairs next to Jacklyn's bed. I was shocked, unable to speak, unable to greet Jacklyn in my usual happy way. I felt disheartened for my poor mother, who was noticeably upset after seeing the baby. I was thankful I'd shielded her from more. The years of worry and loss were now clearly visible on her face. Each wrinkle told me a tale of some hardship she has endured. Her eyes had become small slits. The pain was palpable, and I couldn't change this dreadful situation.

Getting her a glass of water, I attempted to change the mood. She turned to me with a tear in her eye, and all I could do was sit next to her, my arm around her shoulders as we listened to the Disney tune from one of Jacklyn's music boxes—"It's A Small World." Singing some of the lyrics out loud and then turning to my mom, I said, "Everyone has some type of problem." She looked at me, patted her eyes with a tissue, and nodded. I can't remember a day that I'd seen her without a tissue in her hand, thinking about a grandchild who should have been giving her so much joy.

We spent the time with Jacklyn, but now the mood of this visit had drastically changed. It transformed much more for me; it didn't change anything, but it was a revelation. It is something I put aside. The comparison of the other children on this floor hit me. I didn't discuss it with my mom. I had been dismissing it from my own mind with each visit, my armor shielding the awful fact. It was getting harder to depart from reality each time I pressed the elevator button taking me to the Palliative Care floor. Jacklyn was with similar children, each different but, in an unsettling way, the same.

Jacklyn was on the Palliative Care floor, where they aim to manage seriously ill patients' last months. This term was not a familiar one in my vocabulary. I didn't want to know its true meaning. I often received reports that she had a slight temperature. She continued to get pneumonia more frequently. The secretions were bypassing the tracheostomy, even with the cuff. My hopes and high anticipations for this elaborate approach had slowly shattered into a million pieces. For some time, I thought it was working, her problem fixed. I was scared and wanted to scream at the top of my lungs—until I had no voice left. Nothing more to give. Drained. Emptied. But, I can't. Not now, maybe later.

I wish I could have talked to my mother about my daughter's illness. We didn't. All she would say to me was, "Where there is life, there is hope." I would nod but not discuss the details. I wanted to protect her from the grief I was experiencing. Maybe she realized more than she let on and didn't want to upset me—both of us hiding our deepest fears. Collateral pain.

Was it a gift to me that Jacklyn had pleasant features? Would I have adored her less if this hadn't been the case? Would I have hidden in the shadows? I sensed and hated any stares. What would I do if they were frequent? My love would only be stronger, not seeing any abnormality, just differences in abilities. I would absorb the glares and keep all my tears hidden inside my heart while showing her more tenderness and affection. I quietly said a prayer for all the children and their parents on this floor—a prayer that they would not feel different or odd, a prayer for acceptance by others in a world where no one is perfect.

The bag on Jacklyn's feeding pole was almost empty. She was starting to fall asleep as I closed the music box lid to silence her tunes. My mom and I then kissed her gently on the cheek as I tucked the blanket across her chest.

Right before leaving the building, we both went into the chapel. The chapel in St. Mary's had become my daily resting place—a visit, sometimes brief, but still a renewal. It was a sanctuary from my mental, physical, and spiritual pain. We were sitting on the wooden pew next to the altar. I had to resist the overwhelming feeling that I wanted my mother to hold and rock me back and forth, like when I was a baby, with not a care in the world. I struggled against the desire to bury my head into her shoulder and cry. I reminded myself how strong she had been during her life. As I held her hand and noticed the brown age spots and studied the soft, thin creases of skin under her eyes, I gained strength. I was being carried once again, but this time it felt different. He is carrying me. He is rocking me.

Refusing to let my mind go to that dark place was my best defense right now. I could not and would not fall back into the deep dark hole. My daughter needed me more than ever. I repeated to myself that things could be worse. *It could be worse. It could be so much worse.*

It had been a long day, and I returned home to find a message on my answering machine. It was from the Garden City South Parks Department. The handicapped swing would be installed in a few months. October 14 was the date. Sitting in a kitchen chair, I started to cry happy tears. It had been a long time since I'd released those happy, refreshing, joyful type of tears, some reaching my mouth, tasting salty and sweet. A few of them fell from my face, hitting the table. Looking at the happy teardrops, I wanted to preserve them, since I had seen them so infrequently these past ten years.

I could hardly wait for the installation day to arrive. We would be there cheering the workers on. The weather should still be nice enough to take her to the park. I had a smile on my face as my head hit the pillow. Finally, I was looking forward to something positive for her and other special children. It was a small victory for us and other families who don't have the time to advocate for their child.

I slept for a few hours or maybe a few minutes. I woke up crying, shaking. Karl was startled as he came out of a deep sleep. "What happened? What's wrong?" he mumbled. I confessed to him what I'd seen at St. Mary's, what my mom had seen that evening. I spilled out all that I'd been holding inside—what I had tried to bury within me, so I wouldn't upset my mother. He listened attentively, while holding me close. He got me a glass of water, but I continued to try to describe what I found difficult to put into words. "The baby didn't have a face. How could that be, Karl? That baby—that poor infant. On the same floor as Jacklyn. Just down the hall from her. Do you understand they are on the same floor?"

Still holding me, he said, in an almost inaudible voice, "Yes, I know." I was bent over and started to rock from side to side until I was spent, worn out. I twitched with each reoccurring flashback. I couldn't get the images out of my mind. Twitching again, I was afraid to go back to sleep. *How could God do this to an innocent baby? How could he do this to Jacklyn?* I was inconsolable. Slowly a sense of quiet returned; flashes of pictures now included the "Palliative" sign. It wasn't only the baby images. No, not only those images—but the fact they are on the Palliative Care floor—the hospital floor caring for those without a cure, an area where children are placed who are without any hope. I couldn't accept it. Jacklyn didn't belong there. I appeased my inner voice, soothing my mind by thinking she would be moved out of that ward.

"Karl, they will move her off that floor after she is treated and is better." I listened for a reassuring response from him but heard nothing.

Another Child?

It was a quiet night on the Palliative Care floor at St. Mary's. I was there again, visiting, and it was getting late. Clouds floated apart like window curtains in a breeze as the sun was setting. How I wished Jacklyn could see the red and golden hues peeking through the trees from her window. I described it to her, and she appeared to be listening. My desire to be her eyes into the outside world was unwavering. I cherished any alone time that I could spend with her. Many moments cannot be replaced with just a phone call from the floor nurse saying, "All is well." I needed to see and hold her, let her know I am present, have her feel my kisses and hear my voice.

I found myself singing to her in a faint whisper my favorite *Sesame Street* theme tune, "Sunny Day." Nestled against my breast, she fell asleep. I took a deep breath, like a diver right before plunging into the water, as if her scent would fill my lungs and stay with me, sustain me until the next time I visit. Closing my eyes, too, I dozed off for a few moments, content to be with her. She is so innocent and needed all my love and attention. Still, my thoughts drifted.

I could hear my internal clock ticking. Lately it had become so loud that I often found myself starting to daydream, visualizing what the future might have in store if we had another child. I wondered if there would ever be a "second chance"—to hear my baby say that one special word, calling for me, shouting "Momma" while running with outstretched arms. Would there ever be a chance to tickle my child's belly with tummy kisses and hear the endless laughter, a chance to feel those tiny hands and arms hugging my neck and squeezing me tightly? Even a chance to worry—but the type of worry that I had dreamt about. Worry that my child might climb out of its crib. Worry that my child would bruise its knee while running on the playground. Oh, such glorious worries!

Would there ever be a second chance that could allow Jacklyn to hear her own brother or sister's playtime babble while sitting next to her? A chance for me to delight as I witnessed Jacklyn's smile, that soft, sweet little smile she gave when she heard other children's voices. A chance to see the content look on her face as she daintily turns up the corners of her mouth, giving me her very own Mona Lisa smile.

A chance to go back to the toy store where I'd walked up and down the aisles, searching for a special toy that I could buy for Jacklyn—with my heart heavy, knowing she couldn't see or hold any playthings. I'd gone up and down the lanes only to come up empty-handed until I found that one little, curly haired doll with a PRESS HERE sticker, and the mechanical, childlike voice saying "Momma." Oh, not to have any limitations the second time! What a magnificent feeling. I could see myself rolling my cart up and down the aisles, feeling the freedom to buy almost any toy. I would be like other mothers I saw that day who had shopping carts filled to the brim with holiday gifts. Later, I'd watch my baby reach out and grasp the long, floppy ears of the stuffed white rabbit, and curiously shake a colorful rattle or try to place those round plastic rings over the peg.

If we were blessed with a healthy baby girl—the shoes, oh, so many shoes! Shoes to dance in; shoes for church; shoes for the beach; shoes for the pool; pink ones with straps; black shiny ones for that special occasion; gold ones to match a holiday dress. Oh, the endless shoes!!!

"It's lights out soon," the nurse said as she peeked into the room. Surprised by her presence, I opened my eyes and waved her into the room. I needed her help in lifting Jacklyn onto the bed. We managed to do it without waking her. As I took the elevator down to the lobby, my back was throbbing.

Arriving home, I found the various pamphlets regarding adoption agencies and *in vitro* fertilization specialists exactly where I casually left them—on the living room coffee table, the bathroom vanity, the downstairs desk, and the kitchen table. I had hoped Karl would look at them, sparking up a conversation.

After Jacklyn's tenth birthday, I had been secretly researching other opportunities to provide her with a sibling. Months ago, after Karl had left the house to do errands one day, I had called my friend Joan. There was an adoption and fertility conference being held locally that day, and she had voiced interest when we both saw the advertisement in our local paper. As I drove to meet her, my mood changed from excitement to feeling guilty. I was doing this behind Karl's back. This wasn't like me!

Before we entered the conference building, I said, "Joan, you can't mention anything to Karl."

With a concerned look on her face, she replied, "I understand. I won't say anything even when you're sure, because he has to want this just as much as you."

Unfortunately, I hadn't discussed this with Karl. It was never the right time. Many evenings, right before turning off the bedroom lights, I would try to muster up courage but never followed through. Being stressed or tired, or work commitments or another emergency that we had to handle all prevented a serious conversation. Maybe I was just fearful and lacked the nerve.

One night over dinner, I'd tried to get some sense of Karl's feelings. I skirted around the subject. I was anxious that we might be on two different paths. Lord knows we didn't need to have any other disruptions in our relationship. I couldn't bear for us to disagree on this—or anything for that matter. I casually hinted that we should be seeing a fertility doctor or adoption specialist. "Jacklyn should have a sibling," I said softly. I confessed that after Jacklyn's tenth birthday, I had been researching other avenues, so she could have a brother or sister. It felt good to finally get that off my chest.

He was quiet and took a long time before responding. His face looked tired, especially his eyes—not bright blue anymore, but dull and faded. He was holding back, unable or unwilling to answer. Finally, he replied, "I noticed a few pamphlets around the house."

Waiting for more from him, I nervously twirled a small lock of my hair, flipping the strands between my thumb and index finger. I looked intently at him as my chest felt heavy with anticipation. I knew getting emotionally involved with this idea if he wasn't going to agree could turn out to be a devastating blow. But I was already emotionally in too deeply. Karl looked up at me, our eyes met, and I searched in them for an answer. He responded, "Let's talk about this another time." Now, the ice had been broken, my secret from him revealed.

A month went by, and Karl still hadn't made any comments. He had been quiet, distant. As we sat down for dinner one evening, Karl said, "I've been thinking about it." I looked at him as my lower lip trembled. Finally, Karl responded, "Sure, let's do some research on both of those possibilities." I sighed, hearing his approval. Relieved, the tension subsided; every muscle in my body relaxed. Soon, Karl and I were spending many a night discussing these options. Just knowing that we were still a team, planning together and following the same path, removed a huge weight from my shoulders.

During one of our discussions, Karl uttered, "I'm concerned about the physical toll it will take on you if we use the fertility procedures." As we sat on the living room couch, Karl admitted, "I wouldn't want anything to happen to you from all the fertility drugs that are in these booklets." Even though we were not ready to decide either way, it warmed my heart to know he still was thinking of my welfare.

Putting down the pamphlets, I outstretched my hands to caress his straggly beard; then I whispered, "We're running out of time."

Meanwhile, we decided to join the Adoptive Parents Committee (APC) and attend their monthly meetings. The resources available at each meeting helped answer many questions; but most importantly, the discussions gave us a sense of which road we might travel. There were domestic versus international adoptions. Either choice would be a big step, both emotionally and financially. We attended various pre-adoption workshops and social events, some of which welcomed new arrivals.

I was full of admiration when I witnessed the presentation of a couple's newly adopted child. The names of the parents were announced and then the child's name and origin. The audience would cheer and clap, and some shed tears as they walked to the front of the crowd. Standing by a large celebration cake containing the child's name, there would be endless flashes from multiple cameras—almost like a movie star walking the red carpet. To me that was the highlight of each meeting!

The only other moment that came close was at one workshop in which a young adoptee professed her feelings to the packed room. She felt her adoptive parents would always be "Mom" and "Dad" to her. This confession extinguished one of my concerns, and I thanked her for showing such courage and honesty. I thought she was truly a brave young woman to stand before everyone and pour out her heart to strangers. I wondered if our brief conversation and sincere connection was a sign. Yet, right now, I couldn't let my hopes go in any direction. I was scared and frightened because not all the stories we heard had happy endings. There were situations in domestic adoptions in which the birth mother changed her mind and rejected her original promise, taking the baby back and leaving the adoptive family heartbroken. I had to stay opened-minded, stay neutral, and let God lead me down the path He picked for us.

Did God already show me the way? Had I missed a signal? I didn't know. Sometimes I felt so exhausted that I might need more than one sign from him to place me on the correct path. Returning home from that meeting, I could still hear the announcer: "Joe and Jean Smith are here tonight to present their new daughter, Julia Lee, from China."

The Adoptive Parents Committee meetings and workshops moved at a slower pace for us, whereas the fertility doctor's appointment approached in lightning-quick time. I realized that, in our case, we would have to use an egg donor because I was then already in my forties—reminding myself that this fertility treatment was the only way to avoid the same thing that happened to Jacklyn.

Before we entered the reproductive physician's office in New York, I had a sense of loss. I felt less than a woman, less than a wife—not a place I dreamt about creating a family in—and with someone else's egg, too. The handwriting was on the wall, and I was prepared to hear that plan from the doctor. It was the most logical choice. By using a donor's egg, the chance of recurrence would drop dramatically. With despair and failure as a woman continuing to grip my innermost thoughts, I kept those deepest feelings to myself. I pushed them aside, concentrating on the potentially wonderful outcome.

Since I was a devout Catholic, this was a questionable direction. Given our circumstances, I pondered if this was acceptable in the eyes of the church. I desperately hoped so but never made an appointment with a priest. Maybe I was afraid to discuss it, to talk to a priest about how to handle a union joined under God that had a biological break.

We entered the small waiting room in this prestigious New York office, and the receptionist gave us forms to fill out before seeing the doctor. Sitting down, I noticed to my left was a dark-skinned middle-aged woman who was pregnant. I thought that was a good sign. Then, a young, slender lady arrived and sat across from us. She was given paperwork to complete. I started to wonder, *Could the younger woman be a donor?* I was uptight, unable to stay seated for long.

After completing and returning the paperwork to the receptionist, I roamed around the small office, picking up different magazines, looking at a few pages, and then discarding them back to the table. I came across a *PARENT* magazine, opened it and flipped through the publication. After a few pages, there was one advertisement that portrayed a baby sitting up in a seat with a tray table that contained various interactive toys. Clutching it in my hand, it was bittersweet to look at the pictures.

Thankfully, the receptionist opened the door. "Mr. and Mrs. Messina, please come into the office." Entering the office, we sat across from a young, dark-haired physician in a crisp white lab coat. After greeting us and reviewing our folder, he went into detail describing the procedures. I tried to comprehend all but digested only part of his summary. I was just too nervous. There was one thing for sure—my assumption was correct. We needed a donor egg to continue. The last statement from him that jolted me from my seat was, "I'm going to get you pregnant."

A few months passed, and I had completed all the medication and injection cycles. Karl had been a quick learner and gave me all the injections without incident. With the help of an approved egg donor, the date was set for the embryo transfer. The early Sunday appointment came quickly, and we drove into Manhattan. I couldn't shake the thought that someday our contributor might want to know the outcome or get in touch with her child.

Soon after the sedative wore off, Karl and the doctor entered the room. Karl handed me a bouquet of flowers, and the doctor informed me that five embryos had been transferred.

I asked him, "Why were five transferred, and what happens if all take?"

He commented that he could then do "selective reduction." I was horrified! I asked him again because I figured I was clearly still heavily medicated and did not hear him correctly. Once again, he replied, "Selective reduction."

Karl was speechless and continued to stand next to my bedside. Our eyes met, and he saw how alarmed I was after hearing what could happen. While still holding my flowers,

I knew from that moment that there would *not* be another attempt if this failed. Not for me! I felt that failure would be an omen. Maybe with future medical advances, this scenario might change, but I didn't have time on my side.

We left the hospital and drove home. What should have been a happy moment in our lives turned gloomy and bleak. Karl occasionally glanced over and grabbed my hand, but neither of us could muster up a smile. This was not what I had anticipated as I stared at the already wilting red and yellow fallen petals from the bouquet nestled against the dashboard of the car's front window.

Weeks passed, and it became obvious that the procedure had not worked. In an odd twist, whereas most likely anyone who used this science to create a miracle would be upset with its failure, I, on the other hand, was content. I knew deep down in my heart if the transfers resulted in a dangerous number of embryos, I would not consent to selective reduction. How could I make such a life-changing decision that would haunt me forever? Ultimately, I would have opted to keep them all. I hadn't done my homework, and I was to blame.

I was desperate and now ashamed of my poor choices. I hoped for God's forgiveness. Karl was emotionally vested in this, and I'd let him down. I'd let both of us down. Now it was clear that an alternative path had been placed in front of me. I had to pick myself up and follow the new road while praying with each step this time that I'd be guided in the right direction.

Pope John Paul II

We were blowing out eleven candles on Jacklyn's birthday cake. It had been a long day with family and friends. She struggled most of the day, coughing and discharging mucus from her trach tube. It tormented and tortured me to see her suffer, yet I was glad she'd made it to eleven years old. With every cough, we were at her side, to comfort and remove the string-like saliva.

Another milestone reached, and she was almost a teenager. I ran my fingers along her face. It had thinned out, and I admired her high cheek bones. Those chubby baby cheeks were gone. Her eyebrows were thick, and I noticed tiny hairs on her forearms and legs.

It was bedtime, and tomorrow would be the return trip to St. Mary's. As I held her hand, I closed my eyes, seeing the stolen visions that were deep within my heart. She was brushing her cheeks with makeup, as many eleven-year-old girls would have tried to do, with or without consent. Then she was pointing to her legs and asking for assistance to remove the wisps of hair. Next, she would plead with me to shape her thick eyebrows because all the other girls in her class already had their mothers pluck and contour them.

There was no resistance as I continued to hold her limp, yet warm and soft, hand against my face. As I opened my eyes and faced reality, she had fallen asleep. Her hand slipped out of mine, so I pulled up the covers over them before leaving. This had been a slow transformation, yet a cruel trick of nature, because she would forever be my one-month-old baby. I wiped away more drool, gently kissed her cheek, and said, "Jacklyn, you're my big girl, and I love you very much. Good night, my angel."

It had been almost nine months since she'd been admitted into St. Mary's. Update calls during her stay had not been unusual. One morning after Karl and I had finished breakfast, we received a call from her nurse. Jacklyn had been rushed to the emergency room at the children's hospital. My cheery hello changed to a panicked question: "Does she have pneumonia again?" Dropping everything, Karl and I hurried to meet them.

The hospital emergency room had ceased to scare me because of the many years I spent being summoned to what felt like my part-time residence. It had become a way of life, a routine. It was a home away from home. I knew exactly where to go when supplies were needed, and I was even aware of the local restaurants for our meals. Sometimes, I found myself calling the staff by their first names.

A third-floor room had been prepared for her stay, and she fell asleep soon after admittance. "Hello, Cathy. Yes, we're back. Will you be Jacklyn's nurse again?" I shook my head while turning away, not waiting for her reply. I didn't want to be here. Entering the hospital had stopped scaring me, but the way we could leave it petrified me.

Since I was close to home, I left very late that evening to get some needed rest. Tomorrow, October 6, was going to be a special day. I had tickets to see Pope John Paul II.

I tossed and turned all night, with my heart palpitating. I couldn't sleep. I wanted to be with Jacklyn at the hospital. I didn't want to miss anything. It could be placing a cool towel on her forehead if she was warm; changing her diaper because the nurse couldn't get to it until later; playing her favorite music or just kissing her cheek and holding her hand.

Karl assured me that he would stay with her the entire day and into the night. I was sure Karl would be attentive to her. He had done all those things and more, yet I felt lost—misplaced. He urged me to continue with the previously planned arrangements. Weeks ago, I had gotten tickets for myself and two friends. My desire for spiritual guidance and the Pope's blessing made this a golden opportunity. The day was projected as "A Joyful Celebration of God's Family."

It was still dark when the alarm clock woke me. I was meeting Gloria and Jo Ann. But my conscience was laden with guilt for leaving Jacklyn as we entered the church parking lot. We boarded our assigned bus that would take us to Aqueduct Race Track. As I sat in the dimly lit bus, people shuffled by and started taking their seats. The only sounds I heard came from the rustling of paper bags. Most of my fellow travelers were having their store-bought breakfasts. The smell of fresh coffee traveled through the air.

No one was talking, and I welcomed the quiet, so I could think. I questioned myself as to why I was there. I struggled with how I could possibly do this for myself while my child was in the hospital. Unable to calm myself, I shifted back and forth on the cold, hard, plastic bench seat while growing nervous, knowing it was soon time to leave. It was a lot to ask of Karl, too, especially since we had grown accustomed to being a tag team.

I shouldn't have been there—I shouldn't be on this outing with my friends. The thought of possibly having fun and being with my friends just didn't connect. I'd forgotten how it feels. Just like laughter, the real, can't-catch-your-breath type of laughter. It was foreign and had been absent from my life. Now, I was feeling this was a selfish act on my part. Adding to this was embarrassment. After all, I was her mother and should have been with her!

I bolted from my seat and walked off the bus. My friends followed me. Gloria attempted to convince me that attending the Mass was where I should be, where I needed to be. Jo Ann nodded and then added that Jacklyn would want me to go. After telling my friends that I needed a few more minutes alone, they persisted and did not leave my side.

"The bus driver said he was ready to leave soon," Jo Ann said in a shaky voice.

"Go, please go," I insisted. They walked back toward the bus but didn't board it. I could hear them still discussing their next course of action. Again, I yelled, "Please get back on the bus—otherwise you will miss it."

Do I stay, or do I go back home? I needed a sign, something, anything. I walked toward the exit gate. Standing alone in the lot filled with yellow buses, a fine mist created a rainbow over the street lights. The only sound was a slight humming as each bus, one after another, turned on its engine. Otherwise, there was complete stillness. I could vaguely see into each one of them as the interior lights showed images of my fellow travelers. Each bus was filled with eager souls to meet the Pope, each person with a different reason, searching for an answer.

I wasn't looking for much. No, not at all. I was realistic. I didn't expect her to get up from her wheelchair and walk. It wouldn't be too much to ask for her to just become stable: no more pneumonias; to find a permanent facility that is close to home with a caring staff; to see more smiles—just a few more of those infrequent smiles that show me she is content. All this wouldn't be too much to ask for, and if, by chance—oh, such a glorious chance—I could hear "Momma." Just once, only once. Oh, how I still loathe the parents who get to hear "Mommy" and "Daddy" and don't kiss the ground, thanking God for such a gift.

The combination of all the parking lot lights and morning mist brought a bright glow, almost a glistening veil, over the entire parking lot. It twinkled like diamonds, glittering specks in the early morning sky. It appeared as if the Lord had waved his hand over the lot and blanketed us with a radiant, translucent shroud. After seeing this, a feeling of warmth surrounded and calmed me. This was my sign from above, and my insides stopped quivering, replaced with welcome tranquility. I needed to go to this holy place; to be in the presence of the Pope; to pray for Jacklyn and ask that she be freed from her illnesses; to ease my mental pain and accept God's plan.

I realized they were right. Karl, Gloria, and Jo Ann were right. I had to go. Exhaling deeply, I returned to my assigned bus. The door closed behind me as we slowly headed out of the parking lot. My friends smiled and quickly made room for me on the bench seat. As I looked back, I could see one after another as the yellow buses lined the road, hundreds of souls seeking an answer, each different from the next. Each was searching for their own type of miracle—maybe their own peace on Earth.

Within forty-five minutes, busload after busload of faithful followers arrived at Aqueduct Race Track. Thousands upon thousands entered the stadium. Those on crutches and wheelchairs lined the first row along with their caretakers. There were some with baby carriages, and I ached because Jacklyn could not be with me.

As we located our seats, the bright early-morning golden glow illuminated the tremendous green-and-yellow backdrop that was behind the altar. Soon, I heard what sounded like a helicopter off in the distance. I couldn't imagine what a low-flying helicopter would be doing in this area. As it slowly descended, the flags on stage waved, and the surrounding material briskly flapped until the helicopter landed behind the screen. Stillness returned to the crowd. Suddenly Pope John Paul emerged from behind the stage dressed in gleaming white. He was greeted with a thunderous roar. My mouth opened in awe as I clapped until my hands were red. The applause from the thousands of followers in the fully packed arena was continuous until he raised his hands and started to speak.

The service was uplifting for me. Speaking of salvation and how people who walked in darkness had seen a great light, the Holy Father said, "May He free you from all anxiety and strengthen your hearts in his love." Hearing those words gave me some inner peace. I had walked in darkness, yet Jacklyn had opened my eyes to a greater light—a greater, deeper unconditional love, where words were not necessary.

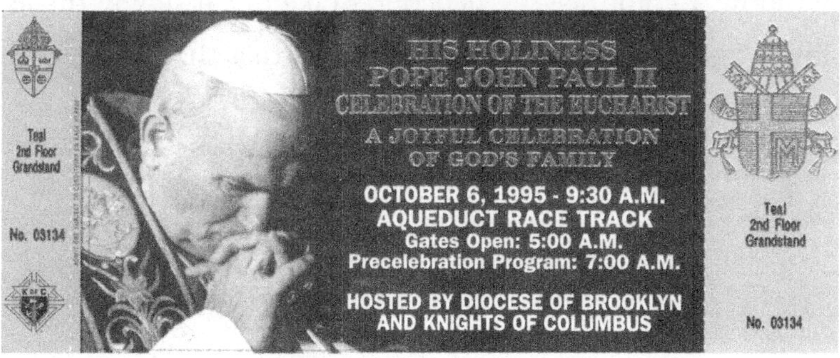
Teal
2nd Floor
Grandstand
No. 03134
HIS HOLINESS
POPE JOHN PAUL II
CELEBRATION OF THE EUCHARIST
A JOYFUL CELEBRATION
OF GOD'S FAMILY
OCTOBER 6, 1995 - 9:30 A.M.
AQUEDUCT RACE TRACK
Gates Open: 5:00 A.M.
Precelebration Program: 7:00 A.M.
HOSTED BY DIOCESE OF BROOKLYN
AND KNIGHTS OF COLUMBUS
Teal
2nd Floor
Grandstand
No. 03134

During the service, he boarded the "Popemobile." You could see Pope John Paul rock from side to side as the driver tried to maneuver the bumpy dirt track. It was way too difficult to continue, and the Holy Father was returned to the stage. How I wished I was seated closer, so I could have greeted him and asked for a special blessing for Jacklyn.

The day ended, and I boarded the bus with my friends for our return trip. It was dusk, an ending of another day, like any other day, never to be regained. For me, dusk is that time of day that is quiet, reflecting only memories kept in the corner of my mind and heart. That day, I gave thanks—for being carried during these past eleven years and for having Jacklyn survive each emergency. Each day had been a gift.

I sat on the same cold, hard, plastic bench seats, but this time I was next to the window. I clasped my hands, leaning forward, resting my forehead against the seat in front of me. Closing my eyes, I wanted to shut out all the chatter coming from each person who passed by my seat. "Please help my child; please save her," I prayed, repeating the same words that had been on my lips the entire day. As I looked out the bus window, I could see the helicopter take off. It slowly turned into a speck in the sky, while I prayed that the Holy Father had heard my request.

October

The gentleman from the hospital's ethical department was following us down the long hospital hallway. I could see him in my peripheral vision. I started to walk faster, leaving Karl as my heart was racing, walking as fast as possible without knocking over nurses and other visitors. As Karl caught up to me, we both entered Jacklyn's room and barely had time to remove our coats before he was standing in the doorway. I remembered this tall, thin, dark-haired man from the ethical department. We met months earlier when Jacklyn had her tracheotomy surgery. I never wanted to run into him again, since for us he was the bearer of distressing news.

His straight-faced proclamation was to the point. "Jacklyn needs to be placed on a respirator permanently." After his blunt statement, I wanted to respond. But, before I could, Jacklyn's pediatrician entered the room and asked to speak to us privately. We had known him since Jacklyn had been born. We followed him down the hallway into a small conference room. His demeanor and ashen complexion alarmed me. I started to hyperventilate, feeling a bit nauseous.

I was in a fog, some sort of trance, and I was trying to snap out of it because I wanted to focus on his every word, shaking my head as if I could rid myself of my protective armor. Still, there was a numbness that persisted. I sat on my hands to stop them from trembling.

"I don't know any better way to say this," he admitted while avoiding looking at us. Karl and I were both staring at him, absorbing every word as he explained in a shaky voice. "The next step for Jacklyn would be to place her on a ventilator. It will breathe for her because her lungs are failing."

I heard our trusted pediatrician. Yes, I'd heard him clearly, and this was probably exactly what the hospital's spokesperson was going to tell us. Our doctor promised to return, leaving the room to give us a few moments of privacy. I found myself pounding the table with my fists. *No! No! They must be wrong!* All these years of fighting to give her the best possible chance had now come to this. *They were wrong.*

"She will bounce back. Leave her alone. Don't have a machine breathe for her!"

As I was looking down at my clenched fists, Karl grabbed my hands. "Let's go home and talk. This is not the place." We got to the parking lot. Leaning against the car, I vomited.

We went home that night, sat at the kitchen table, and poured out our feelings for our daughter's future. We both agreed that being on a respirator was not a cure. It certainly wouldn't give her a better quality of life. Karl mentioned all the negatives. Barely able to speak, he said in a whisper, "A respirator, which isn't pain free, would surely place her in an out-of-state institution, wouldn't change her scoliosis curve, stop fluids entering her lungs, or correct her liver function." Then there was silence—a long, long deafening silence.

I waited and hoped that Karl would come up with another way, another plan. But he only covered his face with his hands. I tried to think of something hopeful, anything to grasp onto for more time. "The positive would be for her to continue living with the use of a machine." That was all I could come up with. But, *living where? For how much longer? How much more pain?* She would exist for us.

Finally, I confessed to Karl, "If it was for me, I wouldn't want to be kept alive by a machine." Then, how could I do this to her? He nodded while holding me close. Patting my eyes, I exclaimed, "God gives and takes life."

Karl said, "Whatever the decision, there should be no regrets. Do you understand me? A change after this decision would not be an option. We could not remove her once she is on the ventilator or bring her back if God takes her as an angel." I nodded, burying my head into his shoulder.

We both tossed and turned all night until I heard the sparrows chirping and was aware of some rays of sunlight peering through the window shades. The tears shed during the night had dried on my pillowcase. I stared up at the ceiling, not moving, not interested in getting up from bed. I didn't want to eat; even water made me vomit. I didn't want to talk; I didn't want to do anything.

I could hear Karl closing the front door as he headed to the hospital to take the first shift. I knew I had to meet him later. Had the time come, the time that I'd seen in my nightmares? I calmed down by thinking of all the instances she'd bounced back, defying the doctor's predictions. She could do it again!

I sat up and saw the little doll on my dresser that I'd bought Jacklyn for her second Christmas to tickle her cheeks and say "Momma" when I pressed the button. I was so optimistic then and thought that doctors could cure everything.

I finally got dressed and left the house, driving a short distance to St. Catherine's church, and sat in the pew thinking, praying, and reflecting about what road must be followed. There was still time. We could change our decision. Wishing for guidance from above to make the right choice and be at peace was all-consuming. Part of me wanted to hang on to our child, to be selfish, and another part yearned to take care of her in a loving way some wouldn't understand—ultimately, to love my child so deeply, so honestly, completely.

I was sitting on the wooden pew, with the light from the stained-glass windows shimmering assorted colors against the marble railing and floor, colors that flickered on my clasped hands. I got up and knelt at the railing, so I could be closer to Mother Mary, admiring her angelic face, praying to her to help another mother who was in pain over her child's future.

The same answer came back to me clearly: I would not want to be on a machine just to exist. How could I do this to her? Would her quality of life be better or continue her torture? Over and over this repeated. I dwelled on the haunting fact that she would be hours away from home—far from home and far from the watchful eye of family. She would be placed where the next available bed was found to fit her enormous medical needs, just a statistic, just a number to fill up a bed, not considering us in the equation. I had to give up, surrender, place this into God's hands. I had to accept *His* plan!

The next day, we informed Jacklyn's pediatrician of our feelings, and he scheduled the hospital's ethics committee to meet with us. As we sat in a private hospital office, waiting to be called into the meeting, Karl turned to me and asked me again how I felt about the use of a machine to breathe for her. "Remember—whatever the decision, there should be no regrets. Do you understand me?"

I searched deep within me, deep within my heart. I knew Karl listed the downward path without saying the awful thoughts we both were feeling. I knew what the right thing was to do, yet, this was a situation I wouldn't want to wish on any family. This was ripping me apart. It was so difficult to say what I thought. Speaking those words out loud to the ethics committee would be the hardest statement I would ever make in my lifetime. Yet, my inner voice continued to direct me: *Do it. Put her into God's hands.*

We were called into a large, dimly lit meeting room. At the opposite side of the long wooden conference table sat Jacklyn's pediatrician, the hospital's ethical representative, and six or more other professionals with notepads. Visually, they were all a blur of dark suits and white shirts. Our doctor started to read all of Jacklyn's medical conditions. We were asked a few questions. The last question he asked was how we personally felt about a respirator intervention.

I looked into Karl's eyes to get a sense of reassurance, his affirmation. After a minute of silence, I attempted to speak. Nothing came out. I couldn't talk while staring at the panel of physicians and hospital representatives. Most were reviewing their paperwork, but a few gazed in our direction. Soon all of them focused and looked intently at us, and I felt all eyes watching me. More silence. My mouth dry, I took a sip of water. I was mouthing words, but my voice was silent. Karl grasped hold of my hand, squeezed it, and then I expressed, "If I were in this situation, I wouldn't want to be kept alive by a machine. I don't want it for her."

As we left the meeting, I was drained but still had a glimmer of hope that she would bounce back. There had been so many years of false alarms. This could be another one. For far too long, we'd been surprised by how resilient she had become over ten years of dodging bullets left and right. This could be another time she surprised the medical professionals. I was scared, just as I'd been in the thousand other scary moments that had become part of my routine. Inhaling deeply until the dizziness left me, I had to remember that I'd told the truth—there was nothing more.

I decided then that it was the best time to go to Jacklyn's room and speak to the head nurse on duty. My request was simple. The day before, I'd received a phone call regarding the playground. I wanted to have Jacklyn released for a few hours to place her on the new handicapped swing that was being installed tomorrow. It was *her* swing, which we had both wanted and fought for so she could fly like a bird. I made my plea but was told that I needed to get clearance from the doctor in charge.

In a brief time, a familiar face appeared. He was a young doctor, and our paths had crossed before. Our frequent hospital visits had become the norm for me, and meeting the same staff was not unusual. Unfortunately, this did not sway his medical opinion. "No," he said. The playground visit could not be allowed. I begged—*begged*—him. He tried, in the sincerest way possible, to explain to me why this would not happen. I clarified in detail the steps that had led to the installation of this swing but to no avail. Deep down in my heart, I knew he was right, but my emotions were riding high. I couldn't see things clearly, nor did I want to. The past week I had been floating in and out of a dream land—none of this was really happening.

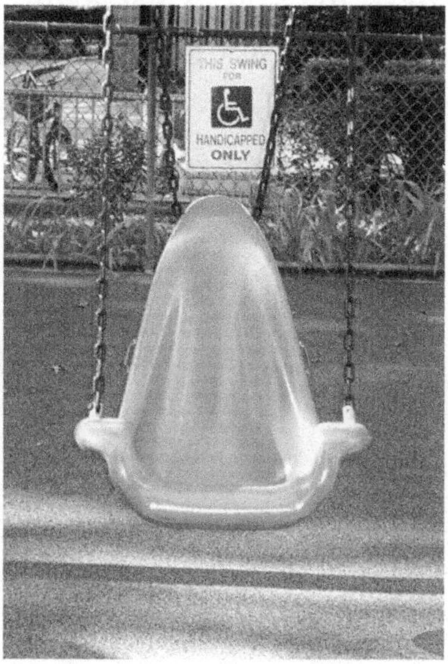

I left the hospital that night wounded, withdrawing from any more negativity. I didn't want to speak to friends or relatives. I couldn't return any calls that were left on our answering machine. As I sat alone at the kitchen table, with my head resting on the tabletop, I thought of a scheme. I considered sneaking her out of the hospital. My plan was to slip out of my house in the middle of the night while Karl was sleeping and take her out of the hospital when no one was watching. I would bring her to the swing and then return her to the hospital. It was possible! After all, this swing was her ticket to be free and fly like a bird!

As I fell into a deep sleep, I could see her swinging through the air, a gentle breeze blowing tiny strands of her hair and a smile on her face.

Free

October 14 started quite early for me. I was getting dressed and planned to be with Jacklyn on this crisp, overcast Saturday, when Karl, who had taken the early morning shift, called. His voice was filled with urgency as he informed me to hurry because she was doing poorly. Petrified, I froze with my hand tightly clutching the phone. Light-headed, I struggled, my memories causing havoc; still, part of me felt she would bounce back. We'd had scares so often in the last eleven years that it was possible. But, another part of me knew this might be it.

I threw on a pair of old jeans and a black tee shirt and ran out the door. Still unsteady, I urgently knocked on my niece's front door a few houses away. My nephew John was home, and I begged, "Please drive me to Jacklyn." As we drove past the tree-lined streets to the hospital, I briefly envisioned Jacklyn's swing being installed at the playground that day. We barely spoke. It was an awkward silence except for John's informing me that he was picking up my mom.

She would stay at his home while waiting for more updates on Jacklyn's condition.

John drove up the circular driveway of the children's hospital main entrance, and I jumped out. I rushed past all the colorful Halloween decorations in the lobby and straight to the elevators on the left. I hurried in before the steel door closed and immediately pressed three on the panel. With my finger still on the button, I was unaware of any other passengers. I pushed it again and again until the elevator reached the third floor. Jacklyn had been moved into a private room across from the nurse's station. I darted past the station and then took a deep breath.

As I grabbed the large silver door handle and opened the door, I could see the sandy-haired resident whom we had seen through the numerous years of hospital visits. He had matured before our eyes from a fresh young man as an intern with a notepad constantly in his hand into a seasoned, and experienced-looking resident. He was standing next to Jacklyn's bedside and was holding a piece of medical equipment over her face. It appeared to be an Ambu[5] bag, and he was squeezing

---

5 A bag valve mask, abbreviated to BVM and sometimes known by the proprietary name Ambu bag or generically as a manual resuscitator or "self-inflating bag," is a handheld device commonly used to provide positive pressure ventilation to patients who are not breathing or not breathing adequately. The device is a required part of resuscitation kits for trained professionals in out-of-hospital settings (such as ambulance crews) and is also frequently used in hospitals as part of standard equipment found on a crash cart, in emergency rooms or other critical-care settings.

Use of manual resuscitators to ventilate a patient is frequently called "bagging" the patient and is regularly necessary in medical emergencies when the patient's breathing is insufficient (respiratory failure) or has ceased completely (respiratory arrest). Use of the manual resuscitator force-feeds air or oxygen into the lungs in order to inflate them under pressure, thus constituting a means to manually provide positive-pressure ventilation. It is used by professional rescuers in preference to mouth-to-mouth ventilation, either directly or through an adjunct such as a pocket mask.

it in a timed matter. All these years, we'd dodged bullets, and she'd survived. Now, seeing my child receive resuscitating bursts of air from him torn me apart. My knees buckling, I nearly collapsed as I grasped onto the bedframe, dragging myself nearer. He removed the Ambu bag from Jacklyn's face and awkwardly left the room without saying a word. Moving closer, she looked so peaceful, a sleeping beauty.

Karl placed her in my arms. He stood over us, caressing her forehead, and holding her hand. During the next few hours two different young residents repeatedly entered the room to check on Jacklyn's vital signs. As I was cradling her, I felt an overwhelming desire to lock myself in the attached restroom to avoid any outside interruptions. I wanted to be left alone, just us three, but could not bring myself to speak or act. My inner voice hollered, *Leave us alone and give us privacy.*" Ultimately I decided that I should not create a scene. They were only doing their jobs. I was satisfied holding her close, smelling her sweetness and kissing her cheeks.

Per Jacklyn's schedule, it was now lunchtime. We asked for the appropriate bag to be hung and attached the food to her g-tube. A new nurse quietly entered, with shoulder-length, jet-black hair. She assisted in placing Jacklyn's g-tube feeding bag on the silver pole that was standing on the right side of the hospital bed. The controls were set, and she calmly asked, in a whisper of a voice, if we needed anything else. I turned and inquired if it was possible to open the window directly behind Jacklyn, so she could hear the birds chirping from nearby trees. She quickly opened the latched window and then left the room. I gave her an appreciative nod before returning to Jacklyn.

Reluctantly I decided it was best to sit in the chair next to her as the pump pushed the mixture of nutrients through the tube and into her stomach. She was content; and, as I looked intently at my precious child, all I could think of was how she'd overcome so many obstacles and proven the doctors' expectations wrong. She was now eleven years old, and they never expected her to live past a few years. Watching her as my tears flowed, I mouthed, "Is this the best that life had to give you?" *Not what I wanted. No, no! Not what should have been for you.*

Hours passed, and Jacklyn was back in my arms again. Her lungs were failing, but her destiny was in God's hands. The residents were continuing their job of monitoring Jacklyn's vital signs. Evening was approaching, and a young female resident with short, dark curly hair entered our room. With her stethoscope in hand, she lingered over Jacklyn for some time. Then she left, only to repeat this scenario.

As I held Jacklyn, cheek to cheek, I turned and kissed her again with the hope that our sleeping beauty would awaken from this evil curse. Karl slowly came over to me and whispered, "I think she is gone." My palm rested on her chest in search of a rhythm. Looking up and shaking my head at him, he placed Jacklyn's hand on my lap. He quietly summoned the young resident, who entered the room with an associate.

After a short amount of time they confirmed, called out the time "4:10 p.m.," and left the room.

I heard this awful deep guttural howl, wailing that was bottomless, a harsh shriek that echoed in the room, erasing all the other equipment noises. Quiet and stillness briefly returned, and I realized all the horrific sounds were coming from me. I cried out, "My baby! My baby!"

Our kind nurse entered the room and was guiding me to place Jacklyn back onto the hospital bed. Everything was happening in slow motion. I was staring at our nurse, who was crying as she left the room to give us privacy. I turned, my hands outstretched to clasp Karl's face. I had *never* seen Karl cry! He was leaning on me and weeping. I didn't believe this was really happening. This was just a dream that had played out in my head for so many years. *Karl, I'm dreaming. I'm dreaming. Please wake me up. Wake me up NOW.* It was the recurring nightmare that I'd experienced almost every night for more than a decade. All those false alarms. Is this really the end? This couldn't be, because a child should never die before their parent.

Jacklyn was gone, free as a bird, her spirit floating out the open window. I whispered into her ear as my tears hit her cheek. "You are free to walk, talk, and see in another world." Yes, I know now that she is free from seizures, pain, braces, and the twisted body in which she was bound.

Time passed, and our nurse quietly entered the room. Tears were rolling down her cheeks as she approached me. I was surprised when she handed me a pair of scissors while pointing to a piece of Jacklyn's hair. I understood her implication and complied. Cutting a small lock of her auburn hair, she took it from my hand, placed it into a plastic bag, and then left the room.

The hospital door remained closed. All the wires had been removed, freeing her as I climbed onto the hospital bed and lay next to my baby. Holding her close to me, smelling her hair, I wanted to fall asleep, too. I wiped away more of my tears that dripped onto her face. My time with her wasn't enough.

Karl was on the opposite side of the bed, with his arms outstretched, holding us both. Soon, with a soft knock on the door, a priest entered the room. He gestured for us to join him in prayer while giving Jacklyn her last rites. I whispered in his direction, "She doesn't need this because she is an angel sent by God."

After the priest left us, I climbed back in bed with Jacklyn. Time passed, and Karl said, "It's time to go."

Speaking in a whisper, I said, "No, I want to stay with her." I pleaded. While hugging us both, Karl gently removed me for the last time. He informed me that his brother Ken was waiting downstairs to drive me home.

"Karl, you'll stay with her?" I asked, as my sister-in-law entered the room to escort me downstairs. As we waited for Ken to drive up the circular driveway of the hospital, I noticed a family leaving with their newborn. Briefly my red, teary eyes met the bright eyes of this new mother, connecting in such a fleeting moment. As we passed each other, I wondered what their future might be, but I was too distraught to really care. She had all the reasons to live, and I'd just lost mine. I entered the waiting car and stared up at that open third-floor window. Open just enough for Jacklyn to hear the birds singing as she floated away.

Arriving home, I barely made it up the steps. I sat frozen on the top step, that initial first step that was always the hardest to overcome with the wheelchair. I didn't want to enter any of the rooms. It was just a house now—*not* a home.

Within minutes, the doorbell rang. It was my friend Joan at our front door, holding a tray of stuffed shells, Italian bread, and a bottle of red wine. Karl arrived within minutes. She kissed us, said she was sorry, and then made us sit down while she prepared our meal. Soon after the table was set and our plates filled, she left, saying, "Eat, and I'll talk to you tomorrow. If you need anything, call me."

Later in the evening, my cousin Catherine called, and I broke the news to her. We spoke for a brief time, and I confessed that I didn't have anything for Jacklyn to wear or for myself. She said to me, "Jacklyn was an angel, and you have something that was made special for her—the pure white crocheted dress."

Upon going to bed that night, I don't recall sleeping. I tossed and turned, moaning and crying for hours: yearning to hear a sound from Jacklyn's room but instead hearing Karl say, "I'm here," while reaching out and pulling me close.

The next day we headed to the funeral parlor. The day had a flat, dull look and feel to everything. Gray, cold—no color, no life! We were instructed to bring the clothing we wanted Jacklyn to wear. I placed the crocheted dress, hair bow, pink tights, slippers, and her diaper into a shopping bag before heading to our appointment. I was numb but forced myself to enter the office. I recognized the funeral director seated behind the desk from the neighborhood. I recalled seeing this stout man with his young daughter at Sunday Mass. *Why, God, does he get to go home and be with his daughter, and I'm here to bury mine?*

I placed the items from the bag onto the table. He grabbed a handkerchief from his jacket pocket and dabbed the droplets on his upper lip and forehead. Looking at Karl and then glancing at me, he paused. He continued to wipe his face. I guess he was unaware that his new client was a child, but then suddenly, I heard a voice in my head yell out, *Diaper!* What was I thinking? For eleven years, I had never left the house without a diaper. As I glanced at this white diaper on top of the other clothing items, I felt just as pale and lifeless. There was nothing left of me. I sat in silence and placed my hand on Jacklyn's final outfit as the funeral director made his presentation.

He spoke to us regarding the time, days, and limos, but I didn't hear every word. It wasn't important to me. We went downstairs to pick out the final item: Jacklyn's coffin. He apologized and said he only had *one* that was appropriate for a young girl. It was white with pink roses at each corner. My mind flashed images back and forth: I was picking out a bright white casket; then I saw myself helping her pick out a long, white wedding gown and a bouquet of pink roses. Fate would never allow me to help Jacklyn pick out her wedding dress. *Oh, all the things that should have been for her and us would never be.* I started to feel sick to my stomach and quickly left the room that was filled with various dark-colored caskets primarily created for adults—only to be reminded that children should not die before their parents.

Black Dress

R*ing, ring.* The phone rang and startled me as I was gazing out of Jacklyn's bedroom window. I sat on her bed and took a deep breath to inhale any of her lingering fragrance. Just being in her room was soothing. "Yes, Mom. I'll take you to see the spot Karl and I picked at the cemetery. I'll be over in thirty minutes. Goodbye." My tears started to soak Jacklyn's pillow where the embroidery of a light pink heart had turned a darker shade. Her sweet smell was still present, not washed away. I inhaled deeply once again before leaving the room.

My mom was ready and waiting at the bottom of the steps. She got into the car and immediately said, "How are you doing? Don't get yourself sick again." I didn't respond. I knew she was a strong woman and had experienced much hardship. She had lost my dad years ago, her only son, and now her granddaughter. It had become clear to me that her ordeals had started to take a toll on her health. I continued to study her pale face, noticing her red eyes; I just nodded as I drove off and onto the Southern State Parkway.

As I entered the cemetery and drove toward the mausoleums, I recalled Jim, a young man in the office who'd helped me yesterday. I wanted a location near a tree, so Jacklyn could hear the birds chirping, and Jim found one site that was perfect. I remember him saying, "I'll wave to her when I drive by."

I followed the curvy road until I saw that tree. I imagined how beautiful it would be during the summer. Then, there would be birds tweeting, an eruption of new life, flying and chirping in their own unique way of communicating. My mother and I walked up the path, my arm around her small shoulders to help support her. She was getting on in years, even a bit frail. I didn't want to lose her. *No! Not my mom, too!* Yet my insides were crying; they were screaming in comparison to the stark stillness that surrounded me.

We sat on the cold stone-slab bench that was adjacent to the mausoleum wall. The silence was interrupted by a single bird that fluttered onto one of the outstretched branches. The black bird stayed for a moment, quiet, cocking its head from side to side as it looked down at us before flying away.

I stared at the blank marble panel that would soon have JACKLYN MESSINA engraved on it. My child's name would be etched in stone forever. I looked at the entire wall. I noticed she had company. Rosemarie, a thirteen-year-old, Andrew, a twenty-year-old; they were all older, but still, she had company.

I told my mom, "She has neighbors."

She replied, "Yes, and she is near Grandpa, too." The truth was that they would spend forever together interred in this massive stone-and-steel building, one by one, row after row.

Token mementos lined the dirt, left by relatives for various occasions. I saw a few flowers as mementos, but it was the unseen ones, the thousand tears shed by the parents of these children, that consumed me. *I was not alone. No, my tears were not alone.* I repeatedly said to my mom as I rocked back and forth, "It wasn't fair. It wasn't fair. Why her? Why us? Where was God when I needed him?" We sat with tissues in our hands, until it started to get dark. Along with the darkness came a hollow feeling that God had abandoned me!

Drained and cold, we left shortly, and I drove on Route 110 until I pulled into a nearby dress shop. My mom needed to use the restroom. While waiting, I started to look at the rows of dresses. I could use a black dress.

Searching and picking out a black dress turned out to be a slower process, because many black dresses were made with parties and happy occasions in mind. Too many beads, shiny, with lace, and low cut. I rejected one after another until I was at the end of the first rack.

Soon a young salesgirl cheerfully approached me and asked, "Do you need any help? What is the occasion?" as she began to explore the adjoining rack. She was bubbly with long, straight brown hair and no makeup. Eager to help me find that perfect outfit, she smiled at me and again asked, "What is the occasion?" *Oh, God—what do I say to her? I hope she walks away. Should I ignore her? Do I lie or tell the truth?*

Since my mother had not returned from the restroom, I continued to shop. *But, what do I say to this young lady? To lie would be to deny Jacklyn's existence. I have become a mother who has lost a child. What should I say?* I didn't answer her and kept rejecting each dress as I quickly pushed them on the long steel silver rod. She was still near. I was uncomfortable but felt compelled to respond. *Why did I have to get a salesgirl who truly wanted to help me?*

Thoughts of what I had become raced around my mind. I wasn't prepared to handle this. What would I say to people in a casual conversation when they ask if I have any children? I wouldn't lie. *I can't now. No, no! I can't now!*

I glanced at this young, sweet salesgirl and paused for a long time; I confessed, "A simple black dress to wear to my daughter's funeral."

Her bright smile instantly disappeared and was replaced with a startled expression. Her rosy cheeks turned ashen, and in a soft, trembling voice, she said, "Oh, no." Then she made an about-face and disappeared through the maze of clothing racks, gone from my sight in seconds.

I wanted to leave as quickly as possible. Swiftly, one by one, I slid each dress down the rod and cast it aside. *Just a few more dresses to view on this last rack—then I'm done,* I thought.

Surprisingly, the next dress was long sleeved, with a round neck, knee length, plain. Absent was any glitter or sparkle. "Good enough," I said while showing my mom, who had joined me and taken a seat on a nearby chair. She nodded, and we headed to the cashier. As I started to exit the store, I tried to find my salesgirl, scanning the store, and even asking the cashier, but she was nowhere to be found.

Momma

It was a chilly October morning on the third day after the funeral. I was in the kitchen having coffee, and my body was still numb. Karl wasn't home, and I couldn't recall when he'd left the house or where he was going.

Now the entire house felt like a museum of objects from bygone days. Formula for her feeding bag was stacked on the counter. The nebulizer and wound-care products were on another part of the counter. Hospital supplies instead of toys were scattered around the kitchen and overflowed into the dining room. Instruction manuals on the feeding pump and a booklet filled with her medication and physical therapy schedules were on the coffee table. The beanbag chair with the wrist rattle we had specially made for her was in the corner of the living room next to her music box. Picking up the music box, I resisted but failed and opened it to hear the chimes of the familiar tune "It's A Small World." It echoed throughout the house, breaking the deafening silence as I held it close to my heart and whispered the lyrics.

I slowly walked down the hallway into Jacklyn's room. I wanted to tidy up her small bedroom, but really, it was an attempt to smell her pillow, blanket, and anything I could find that had her scent on it. My mind drifted and was fantasizing she was away again in the hospital for tests, as she had been so often during her eleven years of life. Jacklyn's oversized bib—which sported a stain I never could remove—was still on her laundry basket. Now, the teddy bear wall decoration we placed there so many years ago, was looking down at me with sad eyes. I could almost hear, "Where is Jacklyn?" Next, I read the poem "Footprints in the Sand" for the millionth time. I focused on the last sentence. "LORD," I pleaded, "I still need you to carry me."

Time passed as I lingered in her room. Opening her dresser drawer, I ran my hand over the folded cotton tee shirts. Next, picking up the small, heart-shaped eyelet pillow I'd used often to position her body, had just enough of Jacklyn's fragrance on it as I held it against my chest. I took deep breaths, inhaling repeatedly, while the pillow soaked up more tears. Eventually, I walked over to read a section of the poem "Heaven's Very Special Child," still trying to accept the role God had asked me to play.

I then walked across the short hallway into the master bedroom entrance. Our bed needed to be made, and I wanted to remove the black dress that I'd worn just the few days ago that was still on the side chair. The little doll with curly brown hair I'd purchased for Jacklyn's Christmas gift was on my dresser. I never brought it to the funeral parlor, nor did I leave it with her. Instead, I gave her the soft white bunny I used to tickle her nose and place her hands around for tactile simulation. This little doll was so small that it could fit in the palm of your hand, but it had tremendous meaning. Through the years, it had become part of our family, and I gave it a permanent place of honor on the right side of my dresser, next to our framed family portrait.

The sun was shining brightly through the peach-colored window curtains that morning. The quilted peach bedspread was in disarray, half on the bed and half on the floor. The house was quiet without any musical toys or medical equipment filling the air with noises that had become so familiar these past eleven years. Nor did I hear Jacklyn struggling with the mucus that would get caught in her trachea. All those sounds were gone forever.

I started to walk between my bed and dresser, where our little doll was perched. Upon taking a few steps, to my disbelief, it said, *"Momma."* I had not touched the button or touched the doll. I immediately stopped, frozen in mid-step, and then fell, collapsing on the edge of the bed. Tears started to roll down my face as I smiled and looked up to heaven. With a quavering voice, I softly said, "Thank you, Jacklyn. Thank you, my angel." I thanked Jacklyn for giving me something she could not physically give to me on Earth, something I'd waited a lifetime to hear. She'd called me *"Momma."*

A quiet calm came over me. Because, from that moment, that exact instant in time, I knew that Jacklyn was fine. A stillness and tranquility flooded my soul, possessing me with an unfamiliar sense of total peace. God's plan was never obvious, but, before long, it became clear. He put us all here for a reason. Jacklyn's mission on Earth was to be "Heaven's Very Special Child."

Assessment

Although this book is about a journey with my daughter, one of the underlying concerns was not having enough facilities to provide adequate care for the pediatric/young adult medically fragile population and their families. This was true more than twenty years ago and, unfortunately, is still true today.

There is a tremendous shortage of beds; in addition, the life expectancy of children with medical fragility continues to improve. Early on, many parents attempt to care for their child at home, but, as the child grows and the parents age, it can become overwhelming. As complications arise, each day becomes more difficult. Just think of giving a small baby a bath and then imagine trying to perform the same feat with an eleven-year-old child and doing it safely. Again, think of a baby in a stroller who becomes a young adult sitting in a full-sized wheelchair. Feeding pumps and ventilators have alarms on them to help prevent a tragedy. They go off many times both day and night on a regular basis. The awakened evening caretakers must be prepared for the unimaginable.

The number of pediatric medically fragile individuals who are younger than twenty-one years of age enrolled in New York State's Medicaid program is estimated at 13,200. This is expected to grow by about 5 percent a year. In New York State, there are only 9 pediatric skilled nursing facilities statewide, which provide 487 beds and only 56 ventilator beds.

Parents will probably visit a few facilities, and that's when they will find out that the population far exceeds the beds available in New York State. The long distance they may have to drive will make it nearly impossible to participate in important doctor visits. Many involve major treatment decisions. An out of state three-hour visit can become a nine-hour ordeal due to traffic and weather conditions. Then, what happens when you get the call that your child is being taken to the emergency room?

I am dismayed and disappointed in New York State and the federal government. They passed the Affordable Care Act and the Americans with Disabilities Act, and they have forgotten about the pediatric medically fragile population.

For all the special children who cannot communicate verbally, don't banish them. Don't send them far away from the only family members who speak *their* language.

The following excerpts were obtained from a report commissioned by St. Mary's Healthcare System for Children in 2016 for the needs within New York State.

Children And Young Adults With Medical Fragility:

A Population Needs Assessment

Executive Summary

Children and young adults with medical fragility are a growing, high-need population in New York State and nationwide. Currently, an estimated 24,000 individuals with medical fragility under age 35 are enrolled in New York State's Medicaid program; this population is estimated to grow at a rate of at least 5 percent per year.

Few providers are suited to meet both the medical and social/developmental needs of young adults with medical fragility; this is particularly true for residential settings. While it is difficult to determine the exact capacity of providers and programs that specialize in serving this population, it may be fewer than 100 total beds statewide. As a result, families experience long waits when seeking needed services, and many are faced with options that are poorly suited for their children. These capacity shortages will only get worse, as life expectancy of children with medical fragility continues to improve and the population of young adults with medical fragility continues to grow.

Background

The challenges for families seeking care for children with medical fragility cannot be overstated. Children typically require a broad range of clinical supports and medical intervention; many require around-the-clock monitoring and care. To meet these needs, families caring for children at home must piece together multiple services and programs—special educational services, home modifications, private-duty nursing services, specialized durable medical equipment—to

Profile of NYS Children and Young Adults with Medical Fragility—Population Profile

Table 1: Total Population with Medical Fragility by Age Group

AGE GROUP	POPULATION COUNT	AGE GROUP AS % OF TOTAL C/YAMF
Total Population with Medical Fragility, Age 0–35	23,800	100%
"Aging Out" MF Population, Age 12–25	9,100	38%
Children with Medical Fragility, Age 0–20	13,200	55%
- Age 0–11 (younger children)	7,700	32%
- Age 12–15 (adolescents)	2,500	11%
- Age 16–17 (adolescents near aging out)	1,200	5%
- Age 18–20 (young adults aging out)	1,800	7%
Young Adults with Medical Fragility, Age 21–35	10,600	44%
- Age 21–25 (young adults recently aged out)	3,600	15%
- Age 26–35 (aged-out young adults)	7,000	29%

supplement the intensive care provided by parents themselves. Even with support, parents caring for children at home typically struggle to manage care responsibilities for their child with medical fragility with demands of work and the care of other children, often with consequences for the financial well-being of the family. For some families, particularly those in urban areas, housing is a barrier; a walk-up apartment with limited space is not accommodating to a child in a wheelchair, let alone more intensive technological needs.

Children and young adults with medical fragility are distributed across New York State, relatively proportional to the total population of Medicaid beneficiaries. Because of their small numbers, in many parts of the state the population is sparse, adding to the challenge of finding age-appropriate services. However, even in densely populated areas, services to meet the needs of the population are in short supply.

Documentation of Existing Services and Service Gaps—Care in Residential Settings

Currently, New York State has a significant number and range of residential treatment providers, serving over 100,000 patients in skilled nursing facilities and as many as 38,000 more in OPWDD certified residential settings with some on-site medical and supportive services.[6] However, appropriate options

---

6 Office of People with Developmental Disabilities, "Report to the Legislature—Residential Request List." February 2016. Accessed 3/13/2016, available at http://http://www.opwdd.ny.gov/opwdd_about/commissioners_page/residential_request_list

for children and young adults are far more limited—less than 500 skilled nursing beds in New York serve the pediatric population. And according to the New York State Department of Health, nursing homes in the state have an overall occupancy rate of 93%, and specialty pediatric nursing home beds are at full capacity, with weekly census averaging 97% occupancy.[7]

Table 4: Number and Capacity of Key Residential Provider Types in New York State

PROVIDER/PROGRAM	NUMBER OF PROVIDERS	CAPACITY (BED COUNT)	PATIENT CENSUS	OCCUPANCY
Skilled Nursing Facilities[8]				
-Standard Residential Beds	618	112,861	104,960	93%
-Pediatric Beds	9	487	472	97%
-Ventilator Beds	54	1,116	1,004	90%
-Pediatric Ventilator Beds	4	56	56	100%
OPWDD Residential Services	371[9]		38,000[10]	11,000 person residential request list

Group residential settings may be more appropriate for children and young adults than an institutional facility, when adequate medical supports are available. However, OPWDD

7 Pediatric beds are facilities or units specifically designed for children under age 21. Children may be housed in general SNF beds that are not specifically identified as pediatric beds.

8 New York State Department of Health, Nursing Home Weekly Bed Census, 1/20/2016. Accessed 1/22/2016, available at https://health.data.ny.gov/Health/Nursing-Home-Weekly-Bed-Census-Last-Submission/izta-vnpq

group homes are also at capacity—the residential request list currently includes 11,000 individuals, with roughly 1/4 indicating that they need residential services within two years. Almost 1,400 (12%) of the individuals on the residential waiting list are young adults age 18–22, and an additional 500 (5%) are children age 0–17.[11]

While group homes may be a desirable option for some families, the typical group-home setting is often ill-equipped to meet the medical needs of children and young adults with medical fragility. While group homes typically do have medical staff on site, they do not have the capacity to serve children and young adults with intensive medical needs at the level that a one-on-one private nurse would. Even if a child theoretically could access private-duty nursing in a family home, currently, regulations[12] prohibit private-duty nurses from caring for their patients in a group-home setting, as their services have historically been believed to be redundant with on-site medical supports.

---

9 Office of People with Developmental Disabilities, Provider Directory. Accessed 1/20/2016, available at http://providerdirectory.opwdd.ny.gov/

10 OPWDD February 2016

11 Manhattan Developmental Disabilities Council, March 2012, "OPWDD Legislative Agenda," available online at http://www.manhattanddcouncil.org/office-for-people-with-developmental-disabilities-opwdd-march-2012

12 Office for People with Developmental Disabilities General Overview Presentation, Changes to Separately Billed Service for People who live in Supervised and Supportive IRAs, CRs, and Family Care Homes, September 2015.

Moreover, in addition to the challenges of finding a placement in the context of this under-supply, when considering residential treatment in either an institutional or a group residential setting, families must weigh whether the environment is suited to their child's social and developmental needs. A skilled nursing facility serving mostly geriatric patients is unlikely to be a suitable placement for a young adult, lacking age-appropriate educational and enrichment activities, or opportunity for social contact with peers.

While New York's nine pediatric nursing homes do provide a vital service as an appropriate setting for many children with medical fragility, they are only equipped to provide services until the age of 21. There are no skilled nursing facilities in New York State specifically designed to serve the young adult, or even non-geriatric adult, population. Pediatric nursing homes face a perpetual challenge of working with families to find placements for young adults aging out of their programs. In the absence of available options, young adults may stay in a pediatric setting past age 20, occupying a bed that was intended for and would otherwise be serving younger children and adolescents.

Conclusion

Children with medical fragility and their families face significant challenges managing a complex combination of medical, social, and developmental needs. While a number of specialty programs and providers offer age-appropriate service options to children, many of these are not available to young adults age 21 and over. As a result, appropriate care for young adults is often difficult or impossible to obtain.

The unique combination of needs that these young adults and their families face requires unique solutions. While a small number of specialty providers and organizations have specialized expertise serving this population, they are currently resourced to serve a fraction of the thousands of young adults with medical fragility in the state. As a result, families experience long waits for needed services, and many must make difficult choices between options that are not well suited for their children's social, developmental, and emotional needs. Moreover, current capacity shortages will only get worse, especially as life expectancy of children with medical fragility continues to improve and the population of young adults with medical fragility continues to grow.

New York State must consider ways to expand service options and capacity of age-appropriate, community-based residential settings serving young adults with medical fragility, and opportunities to ease the transition in programs and services associated with "aging out." Young adults with medical fragility and their families need a range of options, from home care to age-appropriate residential group homes and skilled nursing settings to provide the most appropriate care in the least restrictive setting. Support from the state to increase the number and capacity of suitable programs and providers is the only way to accomplish this goal.

Reflection

As I neared completion of this journey, a writing experience that I pray will help someone, I'm torn as to how I can emotionally explain these past few years. After building a wall to protect myself, it became grueling to chip at each brick, slowly removing each one, to reveal the raw sentiments. Some might say that reliving a painful moment would close the door to that episode—putting it on paper to heal oneself and move on, completing and ending that chapter in your life, reclaiming joy.

Each time I wrote and cried, did I close and seal the door to that memory with Jacklyn? Or, did it open a wound that connected me to her? Was I keeping a cut open, never healing, always alive and present? Painful turmoil that I lived with was my deep connection. Constant worry sprinkled with far too few moments of joy. I'm afraid that revealing and releasing all in this memoir seals the experience and locks it away from me. Could I end up losing the pain and, in turn, losing my connection that I associated with my daughter? Is it possible it could lock her away when the book is closed?

I found it difficult to write about the monster within me, to enter the dark places hidden from the world. Yet, achieving even the smallest of accomplishments gave me hope—if even a small glimmer of hope—that transformed into courage. With faith and love pulling me, helping me stand up when I wanted to crawl, I realized they were always present, silently walking with me at my side. I just had to turn and acknowledge them.

My sincerest wish would be that my experience will help someone. It's up to you to decide what to do with the pain in your life, no matter what it may be, and whether to keep the book opened or closed. I chose to keep mine open as a constant reminder of how faith, love, and devotion carried me. They helped raise me from the depth of darkness to the top of the mountain until I saw the sunrise. Whatever is breaking your heart, don't let it break your soul. Each time you crawl, reach out to pull yourself up, because you are not walking that path alone.

Afterword

We informed the adoption agency that we needed privacy after Jacklyn passed away. Five months had gone by, and I was still despondent but realized that we started down this adoption path for a reason. We wanted her to have a sibling and knew a biological one would be risky.

We were informed the time limit on our adoption paperwork was soon to expire. Attending Adoptive Parents Committee meetings on Long Island was an enormous help in guiding us through the arduous process. The overwhelming stacks of forms that accompanied the effort took years to complete, with our limited time.

A few weeks passed, and our agency contact called, stating she had sent out a packet with information on a baby. Still in mourning over Jacklyn, I had been left in a dismal state. Yet, I knew Jacklyn was now happy in heaven, where she could see, walk, talk, and be free of pain, and this was solace to me. Her gift of calling me "Momma" through the little doll gave me true inner peace. Could hearing "Momma" that day mean something even more? Is it possible she was also telling me to go on with my life and hear "Momma" from her sibling? God does work in mysterious ways.

I still longed to buy little shoes, the styles that a baby girl could use going to church, running on the playground, or dancing in a recital. I longed for a chance to buy a rattle that she could hold and even throw at me when she got mad. I longed for the many things that other parents take for granted.

The new packet arrived, and we immediately viewed the video. There she was, a little Russian beauty, only a few months old trying to get up on her forearms. "Feisty" was the first word out of my mouth. She was a fighter, and that is exactly what you need to be in this world. We made the decision. Our next step was to receive the final packet with *all* the instructions. While we waited for the additional paperwork to arrive, we viewed the thirty-second video a thousand times.

It was a Friday evening after a long work week. I quickly entered the house, weary from checking the mail each day and not receiving that life-changing letter. Karl was already home and downstairs in the den. He yelled up to me to read the agency's letter which was on the kitchen table. He said that I might not want to go through with this adoption after reading it. I paused and held my breath. What could it be?

My shaky hands fumbled through the many pages of instructions. Eventually, I got to the last page. There it was, as plain as could be, the reason he thought I would decline. The document listed: Birth date: September 28th. Jacklyn's birth date was September 25th. Just three days apart. I understood how he perceived it would upset me, but Karl's concern was in vain. With a smile, I instantly realized it was another sign from Jacklyn!!!!

As I sat and continued to look in amazement, I realized how *right* this was. They were twelve years and three days apart. The years represented the Twelve Apostles, and the days represented the Father, Son, and Holy Ghost. I had more than blind faith right in my hands.

Divine direction was now sending us off to Russia.

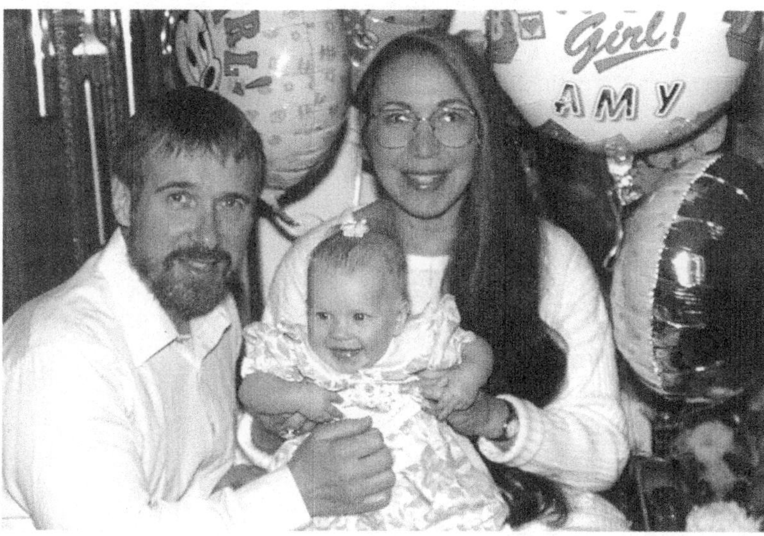

AHRC Nassau

Enriching the lives of people with intellectual and developmental disabilities—www.ahrc.org

Cerebral Palsy Association of Nassau County

Assisting individuals with disabilities since 1948—www.cpnassau.org

St. Mary's Healthcare System for Children

Established in 1870, St. Mary's became New York City's first children's hospital—www.stmaryskids.org

Suicide Hotline

If you or someone you know is considering suicide, please go to suicidepreventionlifeline.org, or call the National Suicide Prevention Lifeline at 1–800–273-TALK (8255)

Adoptive Parents Committee, Inc.

Founded in 1955, APC offers adoption information, support and education—www.adoptiveparents.org

Would you do the author a favor?

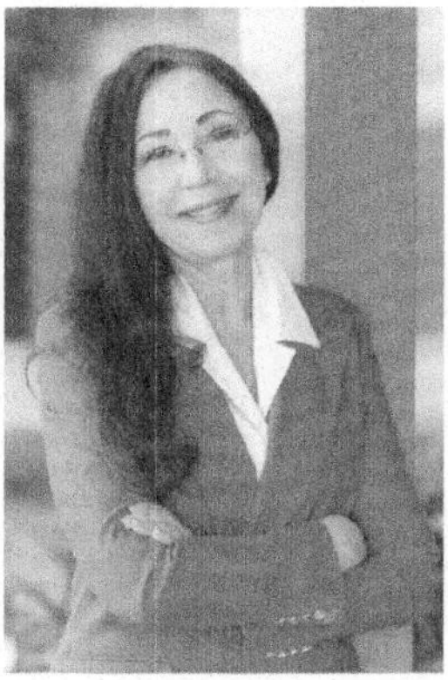

Please contact the author if you were inspired by "*Waiting to hear "Momma."* She would love to hear from you.

Like all authors, she relies on online reviews to encourage future sales. Your opinion is invaluable. Would you take a few moments now to share your assessment of her book at the review sites of your choice (Amazon, Barnes & Noble, etc.)?

Your opinion will help the book marketplace and in turn hopefully reach more of those affected by adversity in their lives, their families and beyond.

Contact:

SpecialChildPressLLC@gmail.com

www.facebook.com/specialchildpress

Thank you very much!

Made in United States
North Haven, CT
20 October 2026

20740129R00184